Neurolo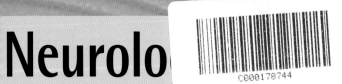

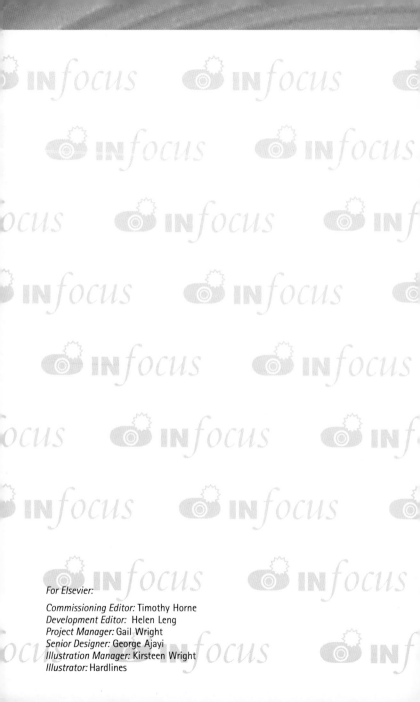

For Elsevier:

Commissioning Editor: Timothy Horne
Development Editor: Helen Leng
Project Manager: Gail Wright
Senior Designer: George Ajayi
Illustration Manager: Kirsteen Wright
Illustrator: Hardlines

Neurology

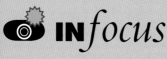 IN *focus*

Michael Swash MD FRCP FRCPath

Emeritus Professor of Neurology
St Bartholomew's and the Royal London School of Medicine and Dentistry
Queen Mary University of London
Honorary Consultant Neurologist
The Royal London Hospital
London, UK

John Jestico BSc MD FRCP

Consultant Neurologist
King George Hospital, Ilford
Honorary Consultant Neurologist
The Royal London Hospital
London, UK

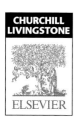

CHURCHILL LIVINGSTONE

ELSEVIER

EDINBURGH LONDON NEW YORK OXFORD PHILADELPHIA ST LOUIS SYDNEY TORONTO 2009

CHURCHILL
LIVINGSTONE
ELSEVIER

© 2009, Elsevier Limited. All rights reserved.

No part of this publication may be reproduced, stored in a retrieval system, or transmitted in any form or by any means, electronic, mechanical, photocopying, recording or otherwise, without the prior permission of the Publishers. Permissions may be sought directly from Elsevier's Health Sciences Rights Department, 1600 John F. Kennedy Boulevard, Suite 1800, Philadelphia, PA 19103-2899, USA: phone: (+1) 215 239 3804; fax: (+1) 215 239 3805; or, e-mail: healthpermissions@elsevier.com. You may also complete your request on-line via the Elsevier homepage (http://www.elsevier.com), by selecting 'Support and contact' and then 'Copyright and Permission'.

First edition 2009

ISBN 978-0-443-10124-3

British Library Cataloguing in Publication Data
A catalogue record for this book is available from the British Library

Library of Congress Cataloging in Publication Data
A catalog record for this book is available from the Library of Congress

Notice
Neither the publisher nor the authors assume any responsibility for any loss or injury and/or damage to persons or property arising out of or related to any use of the material contained in this book. It is the responsibility of the treating practitioner, relying on independent expertise and knowledge of the patient, to determine the best treatment and method of application for the patient.

The Publisher

Printed in China

Preface

The clinical history and the physical examination form cornerstones in the recognition and the diagnosis and management of patients with neurological diseases. This remains true despite the development and availability of increasingly sophisticated methods of patient investigation, since the latter cannot be applied to the management of individual patients unless the underlying clinical problem is fully understood and correctly documented. Ultimately, it is clinical diagnosis that drives appropriate management.

This short pictorial textbook of neurology is intended to help medical students and junior doctors understand and manage patients with neurological problems. In this new series, the text has been updated and new illustrations provided to cover the essentials of diagnosis, investigation and management of the most common or important neurological diseases.

The multiple-choice questions at the end of the book are intended to complement the text, to improve medical practice by instilling further interest and a broader understanding of clinical neurology, and to assist the reader in preparation for both undergraduate and postgraduate clinical examinations.

We thank the two co-authors of earlier versions of this book, Dr Patrick Trend and Professor Christopher Kennard, whose work laid the foundations for this new volume.

Michael Swash and John Jestico
London
2009

Acknowledgements

We are most grateful to our various colleagues, acknowledged in earlier editions, for their help in finding a number of the illustrations used in this book. We also thank Dr Jane Evanson, Consultant Neuroradiologist, who provided some of the illustrations.

Figure 12 is reproduced with permission from Swash M, Glynn M 2007 Hutchison's Clinical Methods, 22nd edn. Churchill Livingstone, Edinburgh.

Contents

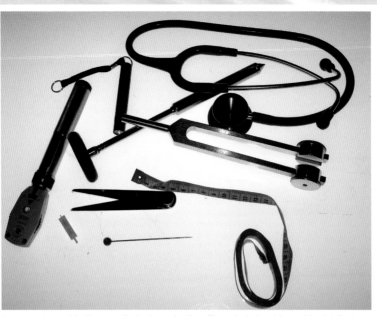

Instruments used in the neurological examination. The red pin head is used in detailed visual field testing by confrontation (see Fig. 1). The two point discriminator is a useful test of fine discriminative sensation, especially in peripheral nerve lesions and in parietal cortical lesions. The tuning fork, used for testing vibration sense, vibrates at 128 Hz. The flashlight tests the pupillary light reflexes, and illuminates the mouth and throat. The patella hammer has a sharp end for testing the plantar responses. The stethoscope is for general use, and also for listening for carotid bruits. The tape measure helps in assessing muscular wasting in the limbs, and measures head circumference, especially in infants.

Cranial nerves I and II

Cranial nerve I: olfactory nerve

The olfactory nerves are part of the brain. Receptor cells in the mucous membrane of the nasal cavity relay to the olfactory tract through the cribriform plate at the base of the frontal skull.

Clinical tests

Present test odours, e.g. oil of wintergreen, or orange essence, to each nostril in turn while the other is occluded. Ask the patient to sniff and identify the odour. Irritant gases, e.g. ammonia, are unsuitable as test substances.

Lesions

Local abnormalities in the nasal cavity and damage to the olfactory nerve fibres, e.g. after head injury, are the main causes of *anosmia*. Other causes include olfactory groove meningiomas and meningitis. The sense of smell is impaired early in the course of Parkinson's disease and often in Alzheimer's dementia.

Cranial nerve II: optic nerve

The optic nerve, like the olfactory nerve, is structurally part of the brain. It transmits visual information from the retina, via the optic chiasm and the lateral geniculate bodies, to the occipital visual centres.

Clinical tests

Test the visual fields as a whole (binocularly) and then in each eye separately by confrontation using your fingers in the four quadrants of the peripheral fields (Fig. 1). This is a sensitive bedside test for field defects, especially hemianopia. Use a red pin head to test for small field defects, especially central scotoma found in multiple sclerosis and optic neuritis. Measure the visual acuity in each eye, using Snellen's chart (Fig. 2) at 6 m (20 ft), and test colour vision with Ishihara's plates. Decreased visual acuity not correctable by refracting lenses or a pinhole is due to lens opacity or to other optical, retinal or optic nerve disease.

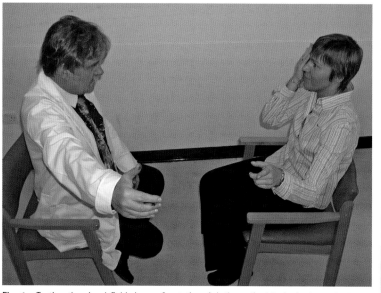

Fig. 1   Testing the visual fields by confrontation. Ask the patient to look at you; test each quadrant monocularly.

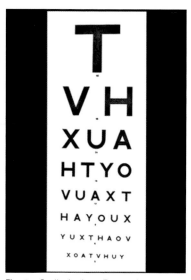

Fig. 2   Snellen's chart. Test each eye separately. At 6 m, which line can the patient read?

Clinical tests

Homonymous hemianopia suggests a lesion in the visual pathway in the opposite hemisphere. Bitemporal hemianopias occur with lesions of the optic chiasm, e.g. pituitary tumour or other suprasellar tumours. Sector defects in the field occur with nerve bundle lesions in the optic nerve or retina, e.g. in glaucoma. Paracentral scotomas occur with demyelination in the optic nerve. Complex field disorders occur with posteriorly located cortical lesions.

Careful ophthalmoscopic examination of the fundus is essential (Fig. 3).

Fundoscopy

A large optic cup (Fig. 4) can be normal but suggests glaucoma, and should lead to measurement of intra-ocular pressure. In glaucoma the optic disc is deep and appears pale (Fig. 5). Medullated nerve fibres (Fig. 6)—sharply demarcated white fibres obscuring the optic disc—are normal variants. The most common abnormalities are due to hypertension (silver wiring, AV nicking, hard exudates, and flame haemorrhages; Fig. 7) and diabetes mellitus (dot haemorrhages, soft exudates, and new vessel formation; Fig. 8).

Optic disc swelling (papilloedema). This is usually a sign of raised intracranial pressure (Fig. 9). It is not associated with visual loss, except at the end stage if left untreated, although enlargement of the blind spot is highly characteristic. Common causes are intracranial mass lesions, e.g. tumours, benign intracranial hypertension, and intracranial venous sinus thrombosis.

Pseudopapilloedema. This is usually due to the presence of small calcified bodies (drusen) at the disc margin (Fig. 10) or to a small optic disc with tortuous peripapillary vessels. This is not associated with raised intracranial pressure.

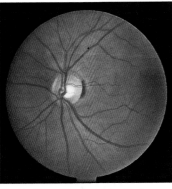

Fig. 3   Normal fundus and optic disc.

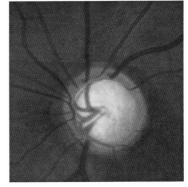

Fig. 4   Large optic cup. May be normal variant or due to glaucoma.

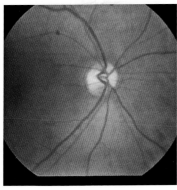

Fig. 5   Deep and pale optic cup in chronic glaucoma.

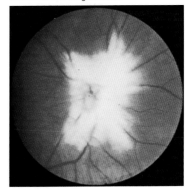

Fig. 6   Medullated retinal nerve fibres.

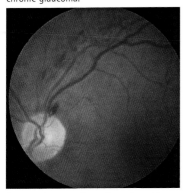

Fig. 7   Hypertensive retinopathy with haemorrhagic exudates.

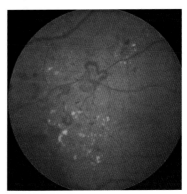

Fig. 8   Diabetic retinopathy; note hard exudates and 'dot haemorrhages'.

Optic neuritis. Local causes of disc oedema are distinguished from papilloedema by visual loss and field defects from the onset. They include inflammation (papillitis), demyelination (optic neuritis and multiple sclerosis) (Fig. 108), vascular lesions (central retinal vein occlusions) (Fig. 11), tumours (optic nerve meningiomas), and infiltrations (e.g. sarcoid and lymphomas).

Optic atrophy. Optic atrophy describes a pale disc. It results primarily from disease of the optic nerve or chiasm. It may be due to multiple sclerosis (Fig. 12), trauma, nerve compression by tumour (which may give rise to optociliary shunts; Fig. 13), neurosyphilis, or toxic causes such as alcohol, tobacco, and medications (e.g. ethambutol). Optic atrophy also follows chronic papilloedema and vasculitis (Fig. 14).

Vascular disturbances
With hypertension, vasculitis or a clotting tendency, the central retinal artery may be occluded (e.g. by embolus) (Fig. 15), or the central retinal vein may thrombose (Fig. 11). Anterior ischaemic optic neuropathy occurs with giant cell arteritis (Fig. 14) but more commonly is atherosclerotic.

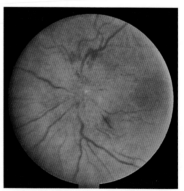

Fig. 9 Papilloedema with retinal haemorrhage due to raised intracranial pressure. The disc is obscured.

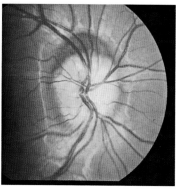

Fig. 10 Pseudopapilloedema, with small refractive bodies at disc margin (drusen).

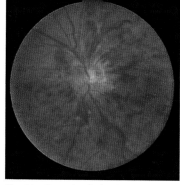

Fig. 11 Central retinal vein occlusion.

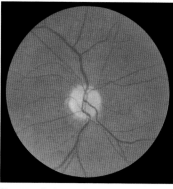

Fig. 12 Optic atrophy; a feature of optic nerve disease or compression.

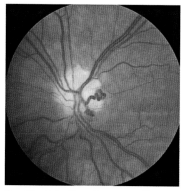

Fig. 13 Optociliary shunts—usually associated with optic nerve meningioma.

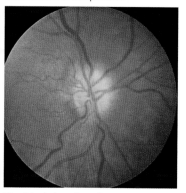

Fig. 14 Ischaemic optic neuropathy due to giant cell arteritis.

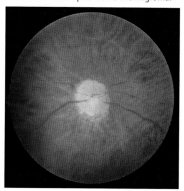

Fig. 15 Central retinal artery occlusion.

Proptosis is abnormal forward displacement of one or both eyes.

The most common cause of proptosis is thyroid eye disease. This may present unilaterally or bilaterally (exophthalmos), often with lid retraction (Fig. 16). Clinical features of thyrotoxicosis are often present, although proptosis may occur in a euthyroid patient. Other causes of unilateral proptosis are:

- *Orbital tumours*: primary tumours such as haemangiomas, dermoids, tumours of the optic nerve (e.g. meningiomas or gliomas) (Fig. 17); or metastatic cancer. An orbital mass will cause non-axial proptosis, with displacement of the globe to one side.
- *Carotid-cavernous fistula* (Fig. 18) is usually due to trauma but rarely occurs spontaneously with rupture of a carotid aneurysm into the cavernous sinus.
- *Idiopathic orbital inflammation* (pseudotumour of the orbit) or *orbital cellulitis.*

Investigations

Orbital MRI is the most useful investigation. This will reveal orbital tumours, or enlargement of the extraocular muscles in dysthyroid eye disease. CT or MR angiography will confirm carotid-cavernous fistula.

Management

Dysthyroid eye disease: treatment of thyrotoxicosis if present; steroids and orbital decompression if the optic nerve is compromised.

Carotid-cavernous fistula: may sometimes spontaneously resolve but usually requires closure by induced thrombosis of the cavernous sinus.

Tumour: surgical excision or focused radiotherapy when possible.

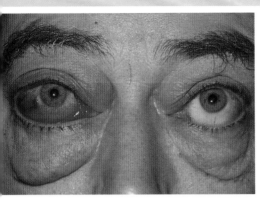

Fig. 16 Thyroid bilateral eye disease, causing proptosis, chemosis and lid oedema.

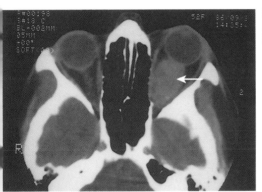

Fig. 17 CT scan showing left optic nerve glioma (arrow).

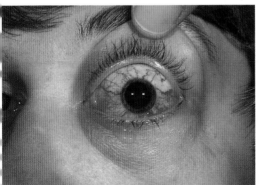

Fig. 18 Proptosis caused by a carotid-cavernous fistula. A loud bruit was heard over the globe. The eye is suffused.

Lesions

Pupil size is modulated by the autonomic nervous system. The pupilloconstrictor fibres are parasympathetic, travelling through the ciliary ganglion. Pupillodilator fibres are sympathetic, arising in the cord at C8, with a long course through the chest and the wall of the carotid artery to reach the eye.

Argyll Robertson pupils
This pupillary abnormality is the classic feature of late syphilitic infection of the central nervous system (Fig. 19). There is slight ptosis. The pupils are small and irregular, with impaired or absent direct light responses, although the near response is intact. Dissociation of the near pupillary responses to light may also occur in diabetes mellitus or with midbrain tumours, but then the pupils are of normal size or dilated.

Horner's syndrome
A lesion in the sympathetic pathway to the pupil is characterized by a small pupil, mild ptosis (Fig. 20), and ipsilateral loss of facial sweating (anhidrosis). The direct light reflex is intact. The cause of a Horner syndrome relates to accompanying signs and symptoms. The most common cause is malignancy. This is usually bronchogenic involving sympathetic fibres at the chest apex (Pancoast's tumour) or breast cancer. Aortic aneurysm causes a left Horner's syndrome. It may also occur in carotid artery occlusion or dissection (with consequent stroke), and in tumours of the base of the skull. In congenital Horner's syndrome the affected pupil is depigmented and appears blue (Fig. 21).

Tonic (Holmes–Adie) pupil
In this syndrome, due to a parasympathetic lesion in the ciliary ganglion, the involved pupil is larger than its fellow and shows a poor or absent light reaction (Fig. 22). Similarly, with accommodative effort, it slowly constricts. When the near reflex is relaxed, the pupil dilates very slowly. This pupillary syndrome is benign and is most common in young women. Adie's syndrome is often associated with diminished deep tendon reflexes, and sometimes with patchy anhidrosis.

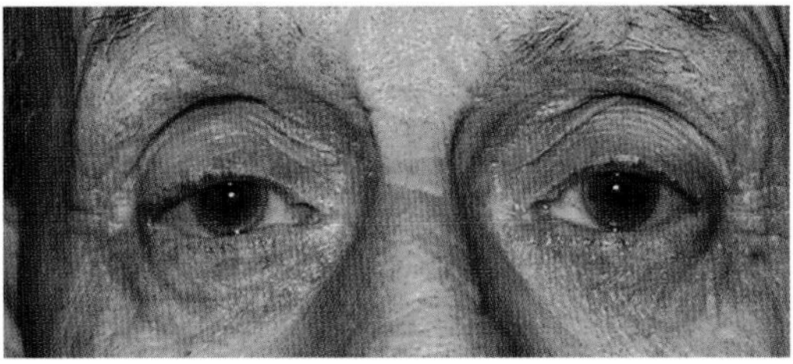

Fig. 19 Argyll Robertson pupils; note the associated ptosis.

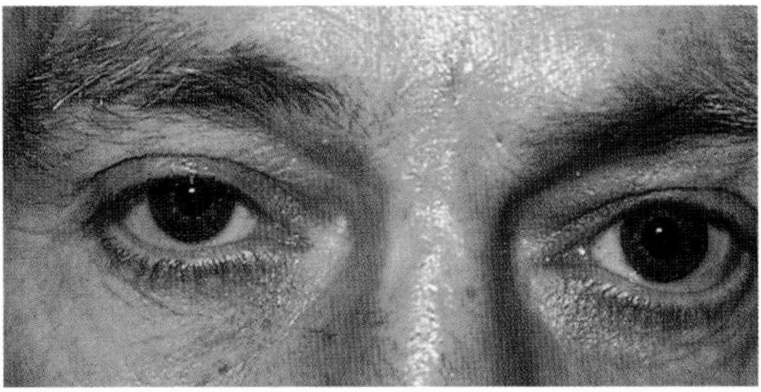

Fig. 20 Horner's syndrome (right). The right pupil is smaller than the left and there is right-sided ptosis.

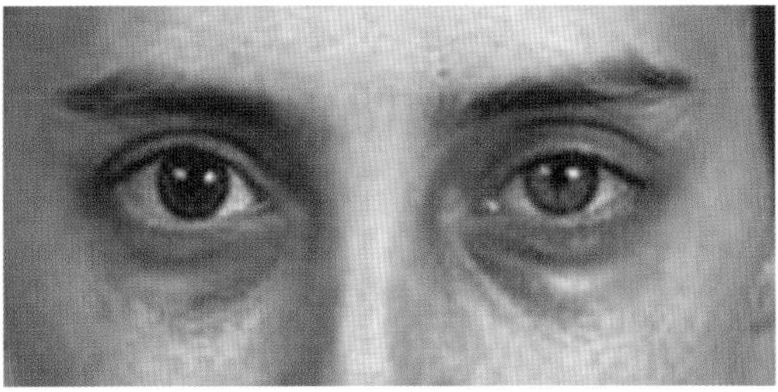

Fig. 21 Congenital left Horner's syndrome. The affected pupil is strikingly depigmented in addition to the signs of Horner's syndrome.

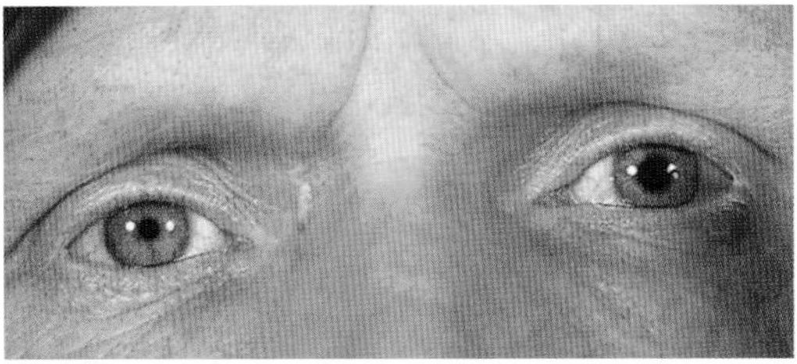

Fig. 22 Tonic (Adie) pupil (left). The dilated pupil fails to respond quickly to light or accommodation.

4 ▷ Cranial nerve III—oculomotor nerve

The oculomotor nerve supplies the levator palpebrae superioris, superior rectus, inferior rectus, medial rectus, and inferior oblique ocular muscles. It also carries the pupilloconstrictor (parasympathetic) fibres.

Clinical signs

A complete third nerve palsy presents with a complete ptosis (Fig. 23), fixed dilated pupil (Fig. 24), and external ocular motor palsy, except for abduction (VI) (Fig. 25).

Lesions

Vascular

Localized midbrain infarction usually also involves pyramidal and cerebellar pathways and results in an oculomotor palsy, contralateral hemiplegia and ipsilateral cerebellar ataxia. In the subarachnoid space, the third nerve lies adjacent to the posterior communicating artery (PCA). A PCA aneurysm, often associated with ipsilateral periorbital pain, is the most common cause of an oculomotor palsy *with* pupillary involvement. Aneurysms in the cavernous sinus involve the fourth, fifth and sixth cranial nerves to varying degrees, in addition to the oculomotor nerve. A sudden-onset, pupil-sparing, third nerve palsy is usually due to infarction of the oculomotor nerve due to atherosclerosis, hypertension or diabetes mellitus rather than aneurysmal compression of the nerve. Arrange angiography to be certain.

Neoplastic

The oculomotor nerve may be involved by cancer, usually metastatic or by direct spread from a nasopharyngeal carcinoma.

Infective

Caused by subacute basal meningitis such as tuberculosis.

Trauma

Head injuries with cerebral swelling or intracranial haematomas may cause transtentorial herniation (coning), compressing the nerve as it passes over the tentorial edge.

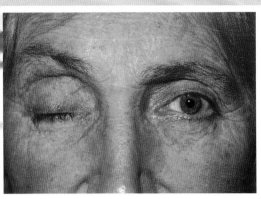

Fig. 23 Third nerve palsy.

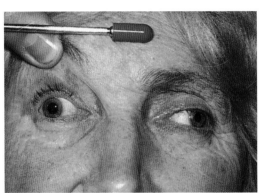

Fig. 24 Third nerve palsy. Dilated right pupil and failure of adduction of the right eye.

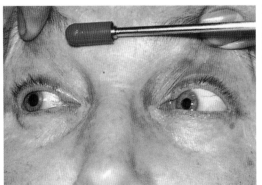

Fig. 25 Third nerve palsy. Normal right abduction reveals normally innervated lateral rectus muscle (sixth nerve).

Cranial nerve IV—trochlear nerve

The fourth cranial nerve innervates the superior oblique muscle. This muscle induces depression and intorsion of the globe in the adducted position.

Lesions

The most common causes for an isolated fourth nerve palsy are head injury, ischaemia associated with atherosclerosis or diabetes mellitus, and cancer of the skull base.

Cranial nerve VI—abducens nerve

The sixth nerve innervates the lateral rectus muscle, which abducts the eye (Figs 26 and 27). It has a particularly long intracranial course.

Lesions

Idiopathic. A surprisingly large proportion of sixth nerve palsies occur without evident cause; they almost all resolve spontaneously in a few weeks.

Congenital. This is rare, due to aplasia of the nucleus or to snagging of the tendon of the lateral rectus muscle in its sheath in the orbit (Duane's syndrome).

Vascular. A sixth nerve lesion when associated with ipsilateral facial palsy and contralateral hemiparesis suggests brainstem infarction. In the cavernous sinus, the sixth nerve may be damaged by carotid-cavernous fistula, by aneurysm of the internal carotid artery or by sinus thrombosis. The third, fourth and fifth cranial nerves are also often involved.

Neoplastic. Tumours of the cavernous sinus and orbital apex, invasion of skull base, and chordomas.

Infective. Middle ear infection spreading to the petrous apex, or meningitis—especially tuberculous.

Demyelinating. As part of multiple sclerosis (Fig. 28).

Trauma. Skull base fractures.

Raised intracranial pressure. May cause a sixth nerve palsy as a 'false localizing sign'.

Mimickers. Isolated ocular motor palsies can be mimicked by thyroid eye disease and myasthenia gravis. Appropriate tests must be performed to exclude these disorders.

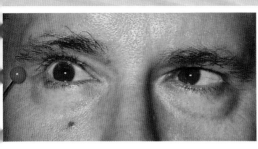

Fig. 26 Gaze to the right shows failed abduction in right sixth nerve palsy.

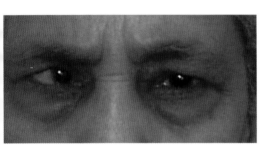

Fig. 27 Sixth nerve palsy.

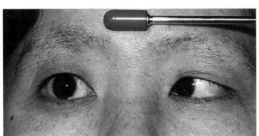

Fig. 28 Failure of abduction of the right eye in abducens nerve palsy caused by multiple sclerosis.

Horizontal gaze palsies

The sixth and third nerve nuclei are interconnected via the medial longitudinal fasciculus (MLF) in order to functionally link the lateral rectus on one side with the medial rectus on the other, and so to facilitate coordinated lateral gaze. A lesion near the abducens nucleus therefore results in an *ipsilateral conjugate gaze palsy*. A lesion in the MLF causes failure of adduction of the ipsilateral eye and nystagmus of the opposite eye in lateral gaze; this is an *internuclear ophthalmoplegia* (INO; Fig. 29).

Clinical tests

Observe the abducting eye during lateral gaze for nystagmus. Always test rapid saccadic horizontal eye movements because in a partial INO slowed adduction, without weakness, may be seen in the eye on the side of the lesion (Fig. 30).

Lesions

Vascular. Pontine infarction, especially in diabetic small vessel disease, is a rare cause of unilateral INO. Lateral gaze palsies occur in lateral pontine infarction, and in major fronto-parietal lesions, e.g. haemorrhage, when the eyes 'look toward the brain lesion'.

Demyelinating. The most common cause; bilateral INOs are frequently seen in multiple sclerosis and are virtually diagnostic of this disorder.

Vertical gaze palsies

Lesions of the neural centres for vertical gaze, which lie in the midbrain rostral to the oculomotor nucleus, usually result in paralysis of up and down gaze. Look for other features of rostral midbrain dysfunction (Parinaud's syndrome), including lid retraction, dilated pupils that react poorly to light, and impaired upward gaze (Fig. 31). Attempted upward gaze may also result in convergence-retraction nystagmus, in which the eyes make converging nystagmoid movements associated with apparent retraction of the globes. The most common causes are decompensated hydrocephalus and pinealoma.

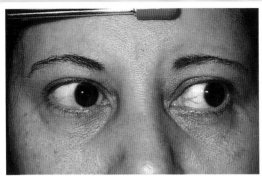

Fig. 29 Right internuclear ophthalmoplegia—impaired adduction of right eye with abducting nystagmus of left eye.

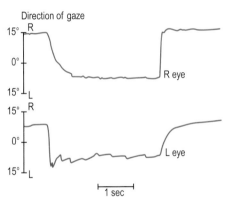

Fig. 30 Eye movement recording of the above patient. Note slowed adduction of the right eye (i.e. during gaze toward the left), with nystagmus of the abducting left eye.

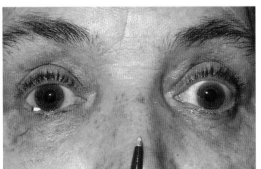

Fig. 31 Failure of upward gaze with lid retraction in Parinaud's syndrome.

The trigeminal nerve is a mixed sensory and motor nerve and is the largest of all the cranial nerves. It conveys sensation from the face and anterior scalp, from the oronasal mucous membranes and teeth, and from the basal dura. It provides the motor supply to the muscles of mastication.

When testing facial sensation with pinprick and touch, remember that the ophthalmic division spreads back to the vertex (the occipital skin is C2), but that the angle of the jaw is supplied by the second cervical dermatome. Pay special attention to the corneal reflex, which should be elicited from its inferolateral quadrant (Fig. 32). Look for wasting of temporalis and masseter muscles, test the power of jaw opening and watch for jaw deviation. Don't forget the jaw jerk.

Lesions

Vascular.   Lateral pontine syndrome (Fig. 33) with posterior inferior cerebellar artery occlusion, aneurysms, arteriovenous malformations (AVMs) or ectasia of the basilar artery in the posterior fossa.

Neoplastic.   Trigeminal neurinoma (Fig. 35), posterior fossa tumours, invasion of the skull base and other tumours in the cerebellopontine angle, cavernous sinus and orbital apex.

Infective.   Middle ear disease spreading to the petrous apex, herpes simplex and herpes zoster infections, usually ophthalmic (Fig. 34).

Demyelinating.   Multiple sclerosis—trigeminal pain is a frequent symptom.

Trauma.   Skull base fractures.

Trigeminal neuralgia (tic douloureux).   Distinctive, brief episodes of severe, lancinating, unilateral, facial pain, usually in either mandibular (mouth/ear) or maxillary (nose/eye) divisions, triggered by touch, shaving, chewing, talking, and yawning. It is slightly more common in women, with onset in the mid 50s, and is usually due to compression of the nerve root by the adjacent superior cerebellar artery. It responds temporarily to carbamazepine. Neurovascular decompression of nerve V in the posterior fossa is the definitive treatment.

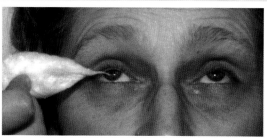

Fig. 32 Testing the corneal reflex. Do not touch the central part of the cornea.

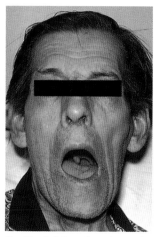

Fig. 33 Left lateral pontine syndrome, resulting in jaw deviation to the left.

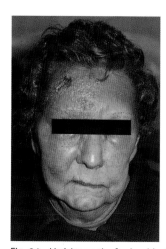

Fig. 34 Vesicles on the forehead in the first division of the right trigeminal nerve due to herpes zoster, a painful condition.

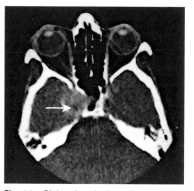

Fig. 35 Right trigeminal neurinoma, as seen on a CT scan (arrow).

8 Cranial nerve VII—facial nerve

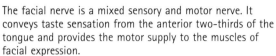

The facial nerve is a mixed sensory and motor nerve. It conveys taste sensation from the anterior two-thirds of the tongue and provides the motor supply to the muscles of facial expression.

The upper half of the face receives bilateral supranuclear innervation; thus, an upper motor neuron lesion principally causes weakness of the lower half of the contralateral face (Fig. 36). A lower motor neuron lesion involves the upper and lower parts of the face equally.

Bell's palsy. The most common cause of facial weakness (Fig. 37). It affects the sexes equally and occurs at all ages. There is acute onset, often with a prodromal ache behind the ear and subjective facial numbness. Hyperacusis and taste impairment may be present in a proximal nerve lesion. Steroids may accelerate recovery if instituted early, and antiviral agents (aciclovir) are also sometimes used. About 80% recover in the first month. In older people recovery is often incomplete. In more severe cases, aberrant regeneration may lead to synkinetic movements of lips during eye closure and vice versa. This may also cause 'crocodile tears' from cross-innervation into the parasympathetic innervation of the parotid gland (from the otic ganglion). Consider sarcoid, lymphoma and Guillain–Barré syndrome if the facial palsy is bilateral. Remember, parotid tumour may cause partial unilateral facial weakness.

Ramsay Hunt syndrome. Herpes zoster infection of the geniculate ganglion causes facial palsy associated with herpetic vesicles in the external auditory meatus and in the oropharynx. Cranial nerves V, VIII and IX may also be involved.

Hemifacial spasm. Writhing, jerky facial contractions usually commence around one eye and then spread (Fig. 38). Spasms are induced by facial movement. It is caused by microvascular compression of the nerve, and by structural lesions, within the posterior fossa at the cerebellopontine angle involving the skull base. It responds to local injections of botulinum toxin into the overactive facial muscle.

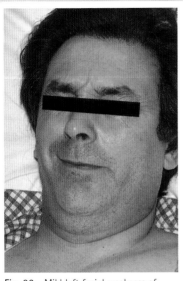

Fig. 36   Mild left facial weakness of upper motor neuron type. Note drooping of the lower face.

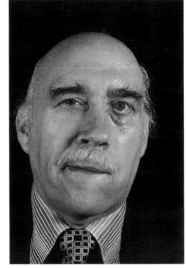

Fig. 37a   Left Bell's palsy. 'Smile' reveals weakness of the entire left face and forehead.

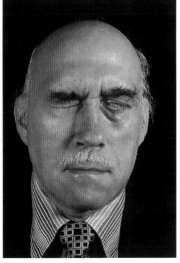

Fig. 37b   Left Bell's palsy: 'screw up your eyes'.

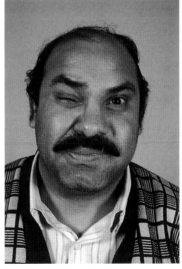

Fig. 38   Right hemifacial spasm.

9 Cranial nerve VIII—vestibulocochlear nerve

Cranial nerve VIII—vestibulocochlear nerve

Cranial nerve VIII is purely sensory and has two parts:

- The *cochlear nerve* (from the organ of Corti) subserves hearing.
- The *vestibular nerve* (from the semicircular canals and otoliths) is concerned with balance and body orientation.

Clinical tests

Test hearing at the bedside by rubbing your fingers together, or by whispering near each ear. Tuning fork tests (Rinne and Weber, with a 512-Hz tuning fork) distinguish conductive deafness due to middle ear disease from sensorineural or nerve deafness. Formal audiometry (Fig. 39), brainstem auditory evoked potentials (Fig. 40) and caloric tests are helpful. MRI of the cerebello-pontine angle is essential (Fig. 41).

Lesions

Nerve deafness may be due to the following:

Acoustic neurinoma. There is progressive, usually unilateral deafness, associated with tinnitus, impaired balance, facial pain or paresis and eventual cerebellar and long tract signs (Fig. 41). Features of neurofibromatosis 1 (NF 1) are often found. If bilateral or familial, consider NF 2 (Fig. 42).

Ménière's disease. Intense bouts of vertigo and vomiting associated with tinnitus and deafness are superimposed on a background of progressive unilateral hearing loss, which often predates the first attack. Onset is usually older than 50 years.

Other causes of deafness. Aminoglycosides, streptomycin and other drugs may cause bilateral deafness. Hypothyroidism may cause deafness. There are many causes of congenital deafness.

Other causes of vertigo: benign positional vertigo (very frequent), acute vestibular neuronitis, vascular disease, multiple sclerosis and temporal lobe epilepsy (rarely).

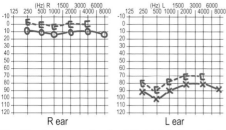

Fig. 39 Audiogram showing left-sided deafness of sensorineural type.

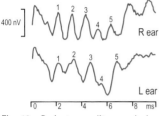

Fig. 40 Brainstem auditory evoked potentials showing left-sided delay of waves 3–5.

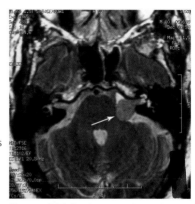

Fig. 41 MRI showing acoustic neurinoma in the left cerebellopontine angle (arrowed).

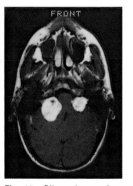
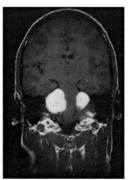

Fig. 42 Bilateral acoustic neurinomas seen on magnetic resonance imaging (MRI) of the brain; axial view (left) and coronal view (right); suggestive of NF 2.

Dizziness and vertigo

By dizziness, most patients mean either vertigo or a feeling of light-headed unsteadiness. With vertigo, there is a sense of motion either of self or of the environment. Once presyncope has been excluded, light-headedness alone rarely is associated with serious neurological disease.

Vertigo, when associated with deafness, usually indicates Ménière's disease or an acoustic neurinoma. Other *peripheral causes* of vertigo alone include acute vestibular neuronitis and benign paroxysmal positional vertigo (BPPV). *Central causes* of vertigo include brainstem stroke (Fig. 43), vertebrobasilar migraine, multiple sclerosis and brainstem tumours. In central vertigo, there are usually other signs to aid localization. Occasionally, vertigo may occur as an aura in temporal lobe epilepsy. Nausea suggests a peripheral lesion.

Light-headedness (presyncope) due to postural hypotension usually develops over some minutes and is associated with fading of vision and hearing. In cardiac dysrhythmias and in carotid sinus hypersensitivity, syncope evolves much more rapidly. A common cause of light-headedness is hyperventilation; this diagnosis is suggested by circumoral and digital tingling.

Testing for BPPV

This disorder is of sudden onset and gradual resolution. Symptoms are posturally related. Reposition the patient from the sitting to supine position with neck extended and head turned to one side. Look for nystagmus and the induction of vertigo (Fig. 44).

Other tests

ECG (Fig. 45) and 24-hour Holter monitoring, audiometry (Fig. 39) and caloric testing, brainstem auditory evoked potentials (Fig. 40), CT and MRI with special emphasis on the skull base and internal auditory meati (Figs 41 and 42).

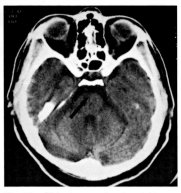

Fig. 43 CT brain scan showing right pontine infarct (arrow).

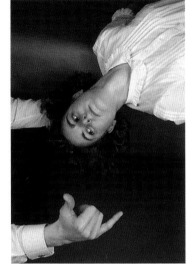

Fig. 44 Testing for positional nystagmus. Note the patient's head is below the horizontal plane.

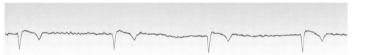

Fig. 45 Complete heart block; ventricular rate 24 beats/min.

The glossopharyngeal (IX) and vagus (X) nerves arise in the medulla and are mixed. The spinal accessory nerve (XI) is purely motor. Nerve IX conveys superficial sensation from the oropharynx and taste sensation from the posterior third of the tongue. It provides parasympathetic innervation to the carotid body. Somatic motor fibres innervate the stylopharyngeus. Secretomotor fibres supply the parotid gland. Nerve X conveys visceral afferents from the aortic arch and respiratory and alimentary tracts. It also supplies sensation to a small area of skin in the ear. Vagal somatic motor fibres supply the larynx, pharynx and palate; visceral cholinergic motor fibres innervate the heart, bronchi and gastrointestinal tract. Nerve XI provides the motor supply to the sternomastoid (Fig. 46) and the upper part of the trapezius muscle.

Clinical tests

Test touch and pain sensation in the oropharynx (IX). Listen for a hoarse voice with coarse cough due to vocal cord paresis (Fig. 47), nasal speech, drooping of the soft palate with uvular deviation, and loss of gag reflex (X). Test for wasting (Fig. 46) and strength of the sternomastoid and trapezius muscles (XI).

Lesions

The IX, X and XI nuclei may be affected within the medulla and upper cervical cord by motor neuron disease, syringomyelia and vascular disease.

These nerves are often involved together in the jugular foramen by neurofibroma, meningioma, granuloma, glomus tumour (Fig. 48), metastatic carcinoma and vertebral artery aneurysm.

X and XI may be damaged in the neck by trauma, usually knife wounds.

The recurrent branch of the vagus nerve may also be affected in the chest by mediastinal tumours, lung cancer and aneurysms of the aortic arch.

Glossopharyngeal neuralgia

Severe lancinating pain resembling that of trigeminal neuralgia is experienced in the throat, especially during swallowing. Carbamazepine is helpful. Consider neurinoma of the nerve, or skull base disease.

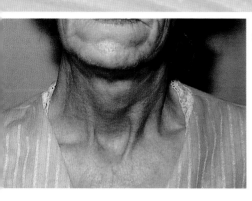

Fig. 46 Wasting of right sternomastoid muscle.

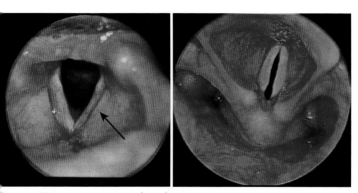

Fig. 47 Right vocal cord paresis (arrow) at laryngoscopy.

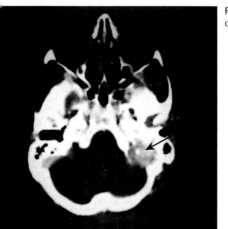

Fig. 48 Left glomus tumour seen on CT brain scan (arrow).

12 Cranial nerve XII—hypoglossal nerve

The hypoglossal nerve (XII) is purely motor. It emerges from the medulla between the pyramid and the olive and exits the skull base through the hypoglossal canal. It innervates the muscles of the tongue, principally the genioglossus.

Clinical features

Wasting and fasciculation of the affected side of the tongue characterize a lower motor neuron lesion (Fig. 49). The tongue deviates to the affected side on protrusion. In upper motor neuron lesions, the tongue is small and spastic and moves only slowly from side to side.

Lesions

Nerve XII is usually damaged in conjunction with other cranial nerves, although rarely it may be affected alone. This occurs in the medial medullary syndrome (in association with a crossed hemiplegia) and in diseases of the skull base, e.g. platybasia, Paget's disease, and neoplastic invasion (usually metastatic; Fig. 48). Extracranial causes include cervical lymphadenopathy (also usually malignant), often with an associated Horner's syndrome. Bilateral fasciculation of the tongue is almost always due to motor neuron disease.

Bulbar palsy
This is the result of lower motor neuron weakness of the muscles supplied by cranial nerves V, VII, IX, X, XI and XII. Features include difficulty in chewing, bifacial weakness and weakness of the muscles of the pharynx and larynx (producing dysphagia and dysphonia), the sternomastoid and trapezii, and the tongue (causing dysarthria). Affected muscles are wasted and, in some disorders, there may be a sensory disturbance in the face and mouth. Causes include poliomyelitis, diphtheria, syringobulbia and motor neuron disease. Videofluoroscopy is a useful investigation (Fig. 50).

Pseudobulbar palsy
Pseudobulbar palsy is due to bilateral upper motor neuron lesions interrupting the corticobulbar pathways. Spastic weakness of the bulbar musculature results, often with emotional lability. The jaw jerk is increased. Causes include multiple strokes, multiple sclerosis, and motor neuron disease (in which there is both UMN and LMN disorder).

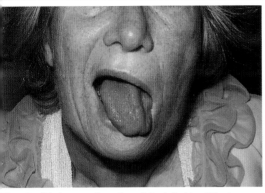

Fig. 49   Weakness and wasting of the left side of the tongue causes it to protrude to the left; caused by XII nerve lesion due to metastatic carcinoma of the skull base.

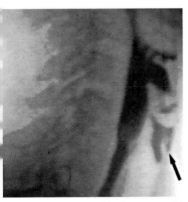

Fig. 50   Bulbar palsy: videofluoroscopy of barium swallow. Note pharyngeal pooling and tracheal aspiration (arrow).

The pattern of presentation and onset is important in suggesting a diagnosis. Disorders such as stroke (Fig. 51) or epilepsy present suddenly (Fig. 52). Degenerative disorders and benign brain or spinal tumours progress very slowly, sometimes over many years (Fig. 53).

Stepwise progression with periods of relative recovery is characteristic of the relapsing-remitting form of multiple sclerosis (Fig. 54). Rapid deterioration may occur in multiple sclerosis. Sudden deterioration may also occur when there is a secondary haemorrhage into an infarct in relation to a malignant brain tumour.

Neurological disorders often develop recognizable stages in their progression, as for example when a length-dependent peripheral neuropathy commences with numbness in the toes and feet and later causes similar symptoms in the hands. Many disorders show late phases of progressive impairment even when the early features have been intermittent; for example, slow progression is common as a late manifestation of relapsing-remitting multiple sclerosis (Fig. 54), and late neuropsychiatric disability may follow severe, unresponsive epilepsy (Fig. 52).

Stroke may present with transient symptoms from which there is apparent full and rapid recovery, but then show a period of disability from which partial recovery may occur (Fig. 55). Recurrent small infarcts cause a stepwise deterioration.

Relapsing demyelinating neuropathies show slow deterioration and slow recovery (Fig. 56).

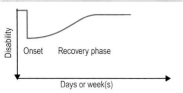

Fig. 51 Tempo of stroke illness; sudden onset and gradual functional improvement or even recovery.

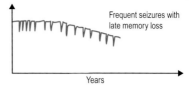

Fig. 52 Tempo of epilepsy: recurrent stereotyped seizure events; with generalized epilepsy there may be the late onset of memory and personality deficit.

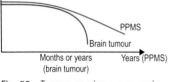

Fig. 53 Tumour or primary progressive multiple sclerosis (PPMS). Intractable gradual progression, accelerating in the case of tumour.

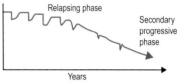

Fig. 54 Relapsing-remitting multiple sclerosis, with later onset secondary progression.

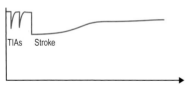

Fig. 55 TIA and stroke; recurrent brief episodes may be followed by a disabling stroke.

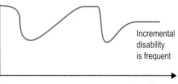

Fig. 56 Relapsing neuropathy (CIDP); phases of progression, often rapid, with gradual recovery.

It is always important to be certain of physical signs, but these, for example the plantar response (Fig. 57), represent abnormality at the time of the examination; only the history describes the tempo of the illness. In many neurodegenerative diseases, e.g. Parkinson's disease, the onset is subtle and the disease is only recognized when disability develops; indeed, this is often pointed out by others.

In spinal cord disease, certain features develop in a recognizable sequence (Fig. 58). With *spinal cord compression*, the first feature is spastic paraparesis, followed by impairment of light touch and position sense and then by loss of pain and temperature sensation. Bladder and bowel functions are impaired later. Pain from root involvement is often a presenting symptom. With *intrinsic cord disease*, e.g. syringomyelia, there is early loss of pain and temperature sensation, with later impairment of corticospinal tract function and of the posterior columns. Bladder and bowel symptoms may be presenting features, and pain, if it occurs, is spinothalamic in type, but often in a local distribution.

Patterns of symptoms and signs may occur that suggest a diagnosis. For example, fasciculation of the tongue suggests motor neuron disease, dysarthria and paraparesis with ocular signs suggests multiple sclerosis, stereotyped motor attacks with altered consciousness suggest epilepsy, and stroke presents with characteristic sudden onset and patterns of deficit. Some of these are shown in the diagrams.

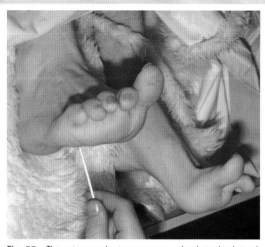

Fig. 57 The extensor plantar response—stimulate the *lateral border of the foot.*

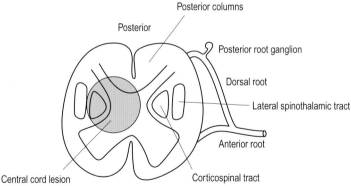

Fig. 58 Localization in intrinsic spinal cord lesion. Note early vulnerability of corticospinal and lateral spinothalamic tracts (UMN weakness and loss of pain and temperature).

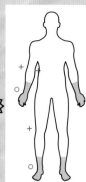

Peripheral neuropathy

Axonal-type peripheral neuropathy with distal weakness and sensory loss

Absent distal reflexes

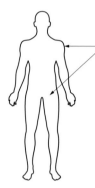

Myopathy

Proximal weakness (hip, shoulder and axial muscles) in most primary muscle diseases

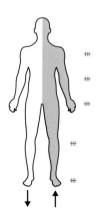

UMN lesion

Hemiplegia with brisk reflexes and extensor plantar response in stroke

Facial involvement

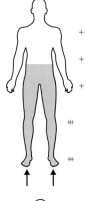

Thoracic cord injury

Paraplegia and sensory loss below lesion level

Extensor plantar response

Sensory loss in *median nerve* lesion to level at wrist on the palmar surface of the hand only

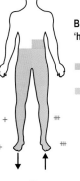

Brown–Séquard 'hemicord' syndrome

- Spinothalamic sensory loss
- Posterior column loss and corticospinal signs

Sensory loss in *ulnar nerve* lesion to level at wrist ventrally and dorsally

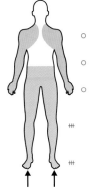

Syringomyelia

Cape-like spinothalamic ('dissociated') loss
Spastic weakness ± posterior column signs in lower limbs/trunk
Pain in upper limbs
Horner's syndrome is frequent
Upper limb reflexes usually absent

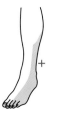

Sensory loss in *lateral popliteal nerve* lesion at level of fibula

Ankle jerk preserved

14 Transient ischaemic attacks

A transient ischaemic attack (TIA) is the sudden onset of a focal neurological deficit (Fig. 55) due to a focal reduction in cerebral blood flow, with recovery in less than 24 h. Most recover in less than 2 h. TIAs are common, with an incidence of 2.2 per 1000 per year in the elderly (>65 years) population. TIA is a variant of 'minor stroke' and may sometimes leave a small infarct in the brain, leading to the gradual accumulation of clinical deficit and dementia with a gait abnormality.

The most common cause of TIA is embolization, either from atheromatous lesions, typically at the carotid bifurcation, or from the heart. Patent foramen ovale and cardiac arrhythmia, e.g. atrial fibrillation, are important treatable causes that should be excluded by clinical examination and investigation.

Clinical features

In a patient presenting with hemiplegia the associated clinical features will point to anterior (carotid) or posterior (vertebrobasilar) circulation dysfunction.

Carotid territory TIAs
These are of two main types:

- *Amaurosis fugax* is an acute, brief, monocular loss of vision. Ophthalmoscopy during an attack may reveal a retinal embolus (Fig. 59). The episode usually lasts 5–30 min, followed by complete return of vision.
- *Involvement of the middle cerebral artery* may lead to weakness and clumsiness, or numbness of the contralateral arm and leg; *involvement of the dominant hemisphere* can cause dysphasia. A monoplegia (arm or leg weakness) suggests a lesion above (rostral to) the level of the internal capsule.

Vertebrobasilar territory TIAs
The most common symptoms are vertigo, diplopia, dysarthria, facial paraesthesias, visual disturbances, bilateral weakness or sensory disturbance, transient ataxia and drop attacks. Cardiac emboli may sometimes also cause skin embolism (Fig. 60).

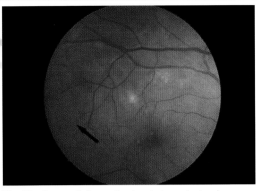

Fig. 59 Amaurosis fugax. Fundus photograph showing a bright cholesterol arterial embolus (arrow).

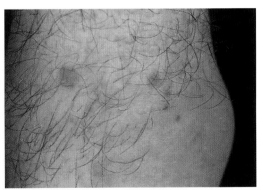

Fig. 60 Purpuric embolic skin lesions from an infected aortic valve.

Investigations

- *Blood tests*: complete blood count, platelets, hypercoagulability evaluation.
- *Electrocardiogram (ECG) (24-hour Holter monitoring) and echocardiogram*: to exclude cardiac dysrhythmia and valvular defect.
- *Doppler ultrasound of the neck*: a sensitive, non-invasive method for detecting carotid artery stenosis.
- *Urgent CT scan of brain* to exclude haemorrhage and to detect early signs of infarction. If possible this should be achieved within 3 h of the onset to allow 'clot-busting' therapy.
- *Cerebral angiography*, using MR or CT methods (Figs 61 and 62), to define any major arterial stenosis or dissection.

Management

For all TIAs daily aspirin 75 mg/day, with a statin and an ACE inhibitor (e.g. ramipril), has been shown to reduce the risk of a subsequent completed stroke. If there is carotid stenosis >70%, carotid arterectomy is indicated. Stenting has also begun to be used. Patent foramen ovale should be closed endoscopically. Hypertension should be managed appropriately, and effective therapy will prevent future strokes. TIAs should almost always be investigated urgently, especially in the absence of a history of any previous stroke or TIA.

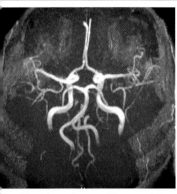

Fig. 61 MR angiogram of intracranial vessels, illustrating the circle of Willis, with the anterior (ICA, MCA, ACA) and posterior cerebral (PCA) circulations.

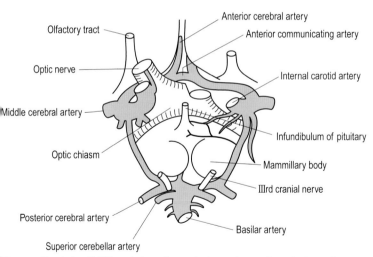

Fig. 62 The circle of Willis and the major cerebral vessels seen from the base of the brain.

The frequency of cerebral infarction increases with age. The overall incidence is 1–2/1000/year. Hypertension, diabetes mellitus, hypercoagulable states, hypercholesterolaemia, smoking and a family history of stroke are important risk factors. There is often evidence of vascular disease in body systems, e.g. angina pectoris or intermittent claudication.

Investigations

Screen for possible risk factors in order to prevent further strokes. Even within <3 h from the onset of symptoms, CT scans can reveal infarction (Fig. 63) and exclude haemorrhage. In younger patients angiography (usually MR angiography) is important and, with MR brain imaging, will detect unusual causes such as arterial dissection (Fig. 64). Lacunar infarcts are often best detected by MRI (Fig. 65). Infarcts within vascular territories suggest embolism (Fig. 66).

Management

If stroke is diagnosed within 3 h of onset, tPA (tissue plasminogen activator) therapy will reduce disability. This requires *immediate* CT scanning and expert reading of the scan. The blood pressure should be monitored but, in general, hypertension should not be urgently lowered because it is often reactive and necessary to maintain cerebral perfusion in the area (ischaemic penumbra) around the infarct. Physical therapy should be instituted as soon as possible to prevent complications such as subluxation of the shoulder, joint contractures, and deep vein thrombosis. Continuation of physical therapy, together with occupational therapy, is important in rehabilitation (Fig. 67).

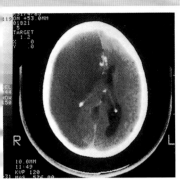

Fig. 63 The infarcted brain is swollen, causing displacement to the opposite (left) side.

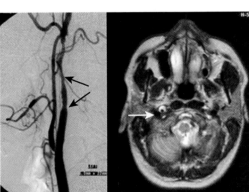

Fig. 64 Right internal carotid artery dissection. Clot in the dissected vessel embolized to the middle cerebral artery (MCA) causing infarction with left hemiplegia. Carotid angiogram shows irregular lumen of affected artery (arrows). MR scan shows crescent of clot in the wall of the carotid in the skull base (arrow).

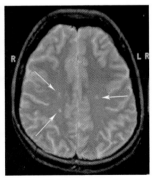

Fig. 65 Multiple lacunar infarcts in deep cerebral white matter (arrows).

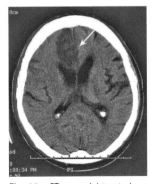

Fig. 66 CT scan: right anterior cerebral artery territory infarction (arrow). Subtle swelling of the anterior right hemisphere with compression of right lateral ventricle and right frontal and Sylvian sulci.

Major carotid (anterior vascular territory) infarction is a catastrophic event. With left-sided middle cerebral artery (MCA) territory lesion aphasia may be profound and persistent, with dense right hemiplegia, hemisensory loss and hemianopia (Fig. 67). Once major infarction has occurred the outlook for recovery is poor. Many strokes, however, are due to 'lacunar disease', small zones of infarction in the deep cerebral white matter and basal ganglia (Fig. 65), or in the pons, interrupting neuronal pathways, especially the corticospinal tracts, ultimately causing pseudobulbar palsy, dementia and incontinence. Since the volume of brain tissue damaged in a single episode of lacunar infarction is small, recovery from a single episode may be nearly complete, but recurrent episodes lead to disability. Acute CT scans, done within the 3-hour window after onset, show subtle changes, usually consisting of effacement of sulci, slight swelling of the involved brain in a vascular territory, and slight low attenuation change. Lacunes are often not detected in early scans.

The circle of Willis (Figs 61, 62 and 68) provides an essential arterial anastomotic system between the vertebrobasilar (posterior) and carotid (anterior) circulations of the brain. This can serve to compensate for stenotic or occlusive disease of major extracranial vessels as well as disease of intracranial vessels. It is susceptible to aneurysm formation at branch points, leading to subarachnoid haemorrhage.

Sometimes an embolus or thrombus can be seen in an intracranial vessel, usually in the MCA or basilar artery, as a high signal opacity in the line of the vessel in an unenhanced CT scan (Fig. 69). Cerebral embolism may be:

- *Cardiac:* chronic atrial fibrillation (due to atherosclerotic or rheumatic heart disease with embolism from thrombus in the atrial appendage), valvular heart disease and atrial myxoma, which, like atrial septal defect, is best detected by echocardiography.
- *Non-cardiac:* includes atherosclerosis of aorta and carotid arteries, and thrombus/platelet, fat, tumour and air embolism.

If a cardiac source is found, anticoagulation is the treatment of choice in preventing further emboli. Initial heparinization, followed by warfarin, is recommended.

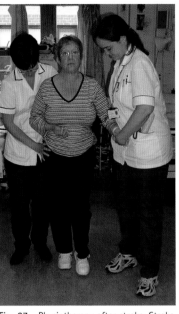

Fig. 67 Physiotherapy after stroke. Stroke prevention is better than stroke.

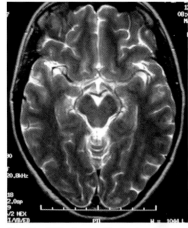

Fig. 68 MRI of normal brain showing circle of Willis and middle cerebral vessels, and the mesencephalon. Compare with Fig. 61.

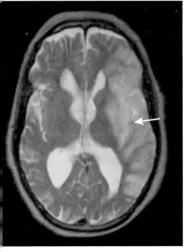

Fig. 69 MRI. Acute embolic cerebral infarction (arrow) due to internal carotid occlusion (left). Signal change in middle cerebral artery distribution, sparing anterior and posterior cerebral artery circulations.

17 | Cerebral haemorrhage

Spontaneous intracerebral haemorrhage is also a cause of stroke. It is associated with hypertensive vascular disease, causing bleeding from hypertensive 'microaneurysms' (Charcot–Bouchard aneurysms) located in deep cerebral structures such as the thalamus, basal ganglia, pons and cerebellum. Substance abuse, especially cocaine and amphetamines, may cause hypertension and intracerebral haemorrhage.

Clinical features

There is a severe headache with progressive hemiplegia and loss of consciousness. The haemorrhage may rupture into the lateral ventricles or into the subarachnoid space; this has a high immediate mortality (Fig. 70). Less severe haemorrhages result in clinical features appropriate to their location; for example, in a thalamic haemorrhage there is contralateral hemiplegia with sensory loss and a disorder of vertical eye movements.

   Although less than 10% of strokes are due to haemorrhage it is important to differentiate intracranial haemorrhage from infarction; this may be difficult on clinical history and examination. CT scanning is sensitive in differentiating between the two conditions (Fig. 71). *Cerebellar haemorrhage* is of particular concern because the patient may initially present with brainstem signs attributed to infarction and later progressively deteriorate due to herniation, brainstem distortion, the development of lower cranial nerve palsies, failure of vital centres leading to death unless the haemorrhage is evacuated.

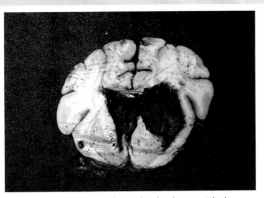

Fig. 70 Postmortem specimen showing intraventricular haemorrhage.

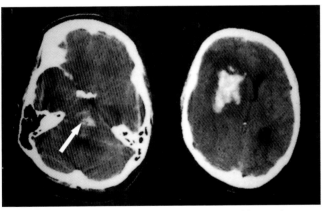

Fig. 71 CT scan. Large right intracerebral haemorrhage with secondary pontine bleed (arrow), due to pressure and hindbrain herniation.

Approximately 5% of acute strokes are due to subarachnoid haemorrhage. It is usually due to rupture of an intracranial 'berry' aneurysm (Fig. 72) but may occur from a cerebral angioma or from rupture of a primary intracerebral haemorrhage into the subarachnoid space. Berry aneurysms are usually located on the circle of Willis (Fig. 72) or at bifurcations of cerebral arteries and are considered to be due to a congenital defect of the media. The initial mortality is about 30%, with a 30% risk of recurrence in survivors in the first week, and then a gradual decline in risk over time. Urgent diagnosis and treatment is therefore essential. Small aneurysms are more likely to bleed than long-standing large aneurysms (>1 cm).

Clinical features

There is sudden severe headache, vomiting and photophobia, often with almost instantaneous loss of consciousness. Examination reveals meningeal signs (e.g. neck stiffness) and sometimes a subhyaloid haemorrhage (Fig. 73). Focal neurological signs may be due to expansion of the aneurysm (e.g. a third nerve palsy with a fixed dilated pupil due to a posterior communicating artery aneurysm), or to an associated intracranial haematoma causing hemiplegia, suggesting a poor prognosis. Hemiplegia may develop also as a result of ischaemia due to cerebral vasospasm associated with the irritant effect of blood in the subarachnoid space. Communicating hydrocephalus is both an acute and a late complication of subarachnoid bleeding due to obstruction of CSF flow in the subarachnoid space and impaired CSF absorption through arachnoid villi.

The diagnosis is confirmed by CT scanning (Fig. 74). Lumbar puncture is unnecessary if the scan is diagnostic. The aneurysm is detected by MR or CT angiography performed urgently (Fig. 75).

Surgical treatment depends on the clinical state of the patient, with conservative management if coma persists. Endovascular aneurysmal occlusion is now the treatment of choice. Neurosurgical clipping of the aneurysm is less often used. In general, urgent treatment is recommended since delay risks rebleeding.

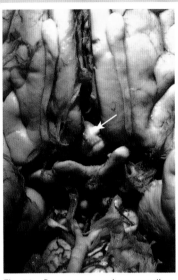

Fig. 72 Postmortem specimen revealing large unruptured anterior communicating artery aneurysm (arrow) between the two cerebral hemispheres.

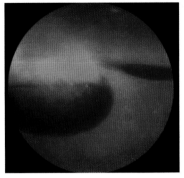

Fig. 73 Subhyaloid haemorrhage. Fundoscopic view after subarachnoid haemorrhage.

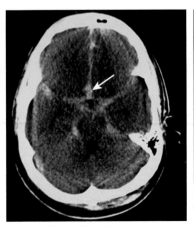

Fig. 74 CT scan. There is extensive subarachnoid blood in the basal cisterns; an anterior communicating aneurysm is suspected (arrow).

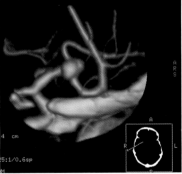

Fig. 75 CT angiogram. Aneurysm of anterior communicating artery (centre of image).

Giant carotid aneurysm

This presents in late middle life with headache, visual field defects, but less often with haemorrhage. Giant aneurysms are larger than 15 mm in diameter (Fig. 76).

Giant basilar aneurysm

Tortuous fusiform aneurysmal enlargement of the basilar artery may cause cranial nerve palsies, or trigeminal pain. Aneurysms located at the tip of the basilar artery may reach giant proportions (>1 cm diameter) and may bleed or thrombose.

Staging subarachnoid haemorrhage

This staging system (Fig. 77) is useful for estimating the prognosis after subarachnoid bleeding.

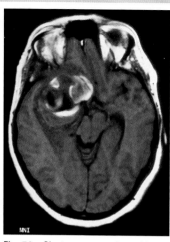

Fig. 76 Giant aneurysm of carotid artery, partially thrombosed. Clot appears white, and the lumen is dark.

Grade		Mortality (%)
I	Asymptomatic	11%
II	Severe headache but no neurologic deficit other than a cranial nerve palsy	26%
III	Headache with drowsiness or mild deficit	33%
IV	Headache with stupor, moderate to severe hemiparesis, and possible early rigidity and vegetative disturbances	71%
V	Deep coma, decorticate rigidity and a moribund appearance	100%

Fig. 77 Staging of subarachnoid haemorrhage.

Developmental abnormalities can cause abnormal connections between the arterial and venous systems. AVMs vary in size, tend to expand over years, and can occur anywhere within the brain or spinal cord, as in other organs.

Clinical features

AVMs present at any age with haemorrhage. They also cause focal seizures. Rupture usually leads to both subarachnoid and intracerebral haemorrhage, with focal neurological deficits or coma. The consequences of rupture are not as severe as after berry aneurysm rupture, the mortality being about 10%. The risk of haemorrhage of unruptured AVMs is about 3% per year.

Management

The diagnosis is confirmed by MR imaging (Fig. 78), and the feeding vessels determined by MR or CT angiography (Fig. 80). Neurovascular procedures aimed at occluding the malformation include embolization therapy and stereotactic radiotherapy.

Cavernous haemangiomas

These are small angiomas (Fig. 79), of venous rather than arterial origin, which present with stroke-like episodes due to local haemorrhage, or with epilepsy. They are sometimes familial and are often found incidentally in MR scans done for another indication.

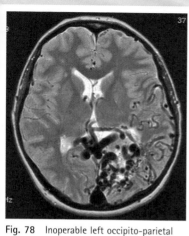

Fig. 78 Inoperable left occipito-parietal AVM with multiple draining and feeding vessels. Several associated aneurysms are seen as rounded dark zones posteriorly.

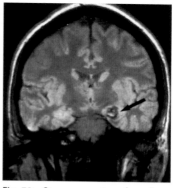

Fig. 79 Cavernous angioma (arrow) revealed on an MRI scan in medial aspect of right temporal lobe. This patient presented with epilepsy.

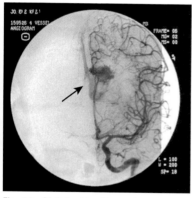

Fig. 80 Digital subtraction angiogram revealing frontal AVM arising from anterior cerebral artery circulation (arrow).

In adults, brain tumours represent 2% of all malignancies. Half are primary tumours of the brain, its coverings, and the pituitary gland; the other half are metastases. Certain genetic disorders (e.g. neurofibromatosis) predispose to brain tumours.

Clinical features

Brain tumours usually present with progressive focal symptoms and signs. Presentation solely with features of raised intracranial pressure is unusual. Posterior fossa tumours, however, may cause obstructive hydrocephalus, leading to headache and vomiting. Partial or generalized epilepsy is especially frequent with frontal and temporal tumours, or tumours involving cerebral cortex (Fig. 81), often without objective abnormality on clinical examination. A seizure disorder commencing after adolescence should always raise suspicion of brain tumour. About 10% of patients with epilepsy commencing after age 20 years have brain tumours, especially astrocytoma (Figs 81 and 82), metastases (Fig. 83) or lymphoma (Fig. 84). Large, slowly growing tumours (Fig. 85), e.g. frontal meningiomas, cause progressive mental slowing, forgetfulness and personality change. Left-sided cerebral tumours lead to a progressive language disturbance (aphasia) that may be mistaken for dementia, either with focal disturbances or raised intracranial pressure. Headache is a surprisingly infrequent presentation.

A combination of progressive partial seizures (often with secondary generalization) and focal signs (especially subtle aphasia, corticospinal signs and hemianopia), with morning headache is characteristic of supratentorial tumours. Sometimes the progressive course is punctuated by sudden stroke-like episodes due to infarction or haemorrhage in a malignant tumour. Papilloedema is a useful but rather uncommon sign that indicates severe raised intracranial pressure. Malignant gliomas may spread across the corpus callosum to the contralateral hemisphere. They often have a cystic appearance on CT or MR images; the prognosis of Grade 4 gliomas is very poor, but benign (Grade 1) gliomas are compatible with survival for many years.

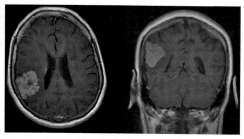

Fig. 81 MRI Right parietal glioma. There is some compression of the lateral ventricle.

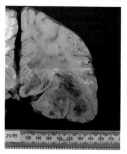

Fig. 82 Glioma of left temporal lobe with swelling of left hemisphere, at autopsy. Note the oedema with obliteration of sulci.

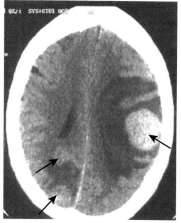

Fig. 83 CT: multiple metastases in both hemispheres (arrows). There is marked oedema.

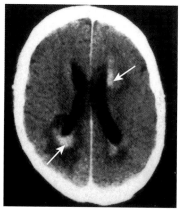

Fig. 84 CT: lymphoma with multiple lesions in the deep white matter (arrows).

Lesions

Gliomas: intrinsic neuroepithelial tumours arising from the glia (supporting tissue of the brain). They are locally invasive and may be cystic; they are often highly malignant, and low grade gliomas may undergo malignant transformation later in their course.

Astrocytomas: in the corpus callosum produce marked personality changes, with frontal lobe deficits. The temporal lobe (Fig. 82) is a common location of astrocytomas, often causing partial seizures with a prominent olfactory and gustatory aura. The focal mass lesion may lead to uncal herniation, causing drowsiness and ipsilateral third nerve palsy.

Lymphoma: (Fig. 84) occurs as a primary tumour or as part of a generalized process. It is especially common in acquired immune deficiency syndrome (AIDS).

Metastases: (Fig. 83) frequently multiple and usually located at the grey/white matter junction. Tumours of the lung, breast, kidney and thyroid, as well as melanomas, are common primary tumours.

Meningiomas: (Figs 85 and 86) common tumours, usually located at the convexity of the brain, on the sphenoid wing, in the parasellar region, in the lateral ventricles, in the posterior fossa or in the orbit. They are slow growing and may be very large, causing a stroke-like presentation or leading to recurrent focal or generalized seizures. Sometimes, small cortical meningiomas may present with epilepsy. If technically feasible, surgical removal should be complete. Incidental meningiomas are found in up to 4% of people at autopsy.

Colloid cysts: (Fig. 87) dense cystic tumours containing proteinaceous fluid, usually found in the third ventricle. They may lead to headache or sudden brief loss of consciousness, due to intermittent hydrocephalus.

Medulloblastoma: (Fig. 88) a malignant tumour of childhood, sensitive to radiation and chemotherapy, usually found in the cerebellum, that may metastasize widely within the cerebrospinal fluid (CSF) pathways.

Schwannomas: non-malignant but locally invasive tumours usually arising from cranial nerve VIII (Fig. 40).

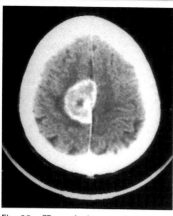

Fig. 85 CT: meningioma at the convexity.

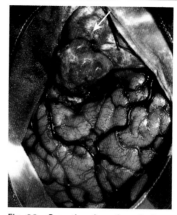

Fig. 86 Operative view of meningioma on parietal surface of brain (arrow).

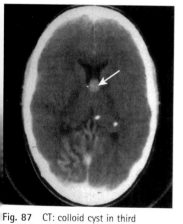

Fig. 87 CT: colloid cyst in third ventricle, appearing as a high-density lesion (arrow). There is infarction in the right occipital region with hyperperfusion of the ischaemic region.

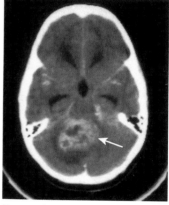

Fig. 88 CT: medulloblastoma in vermis of cerebellum of a child (arrow).

Pituitary tumours

Pituitary adenomas may be functioning or non-functioning. They may present with mass effects on neighbouring structures. They are rarely malignant.

Large tumours erode the pituitary fossa (Fig. 89) and damage the optic chiasm, leading to bitemporal hemianopia, optic atrophy and panhypopituitarism. Functioning tumours are usually small, especially prolactinomas, which cause infertility, loss of libido and galactorrhoea with amenorrhoea. Acromegaly (Fig. 90) occurs when there is uncontrolled secretion of growth hormone, and Cushing's syndrome when there is secretion of ACTH. Large tumours or those involving the hypothalamus cause diabetes insipidus and loss of gonadotrophic hormones. CT and MRI scanning accurately delineate the pituitary fossa and the extent of lateral and superior growth of pituitary tumours (Fig. 91). Surgical excision is usually indicated although some adenomas, especially prolactinomas, can be managed medically.

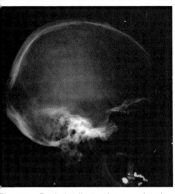

Fig. 89 Eroded sella turcica associated with large chromophobe adenoma of pituitary.

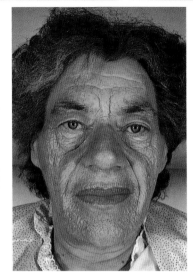

Fig. 90 Acromegaly.

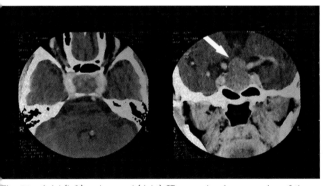

Fig. 91 Axial (left) and coronal (right) CT scans showing expansion of the pituitary fossa by a tumour. Note the suprasellar extension (arrow).

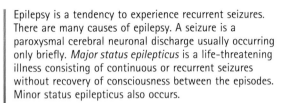

21 Epilepsy

Epilepsy

Epilepsy is a tendency to experience recurrent seizures. There are many causes of epilepsy. A seizure is a paroxysmal cerebral neuronal discharge usually occurring only briefly. *Major status epilepticus* is a life-threatening illness consisting of continuous or recurrent seizures without recovery of consciousness between the episodes. Minor status epilepticus also occurs.

Classification

Generalized epilepsy: without focal onset

Tonic/clonic (major generalized) attacks: begin with a cry, transient limb stiffening and bodily jerking. The attack usually concludes in a few minutes. Tongue biting and incontinence may occur. Typically, the patient experiences postictal drowsiness.

Absence (minor generalized) attacks: brief blank staring spells with dilated pupils, eyelid fluttering, facial and limb jerks, fumbling of the hands. The electroencephalogram (EEG) is characteristic with three-per-second high-voltage spike and wave discharges (Fig. 92). Myoclonus (brief jerks, either focal or generalized) is a frequent feature of idiopathic epilepsy.

Partial (focal or localization–related) epilepsy: with focal onset

a) Simple (without altered consciousness): may be motor (adversive or a Jacksonian march), sensory (visual, auditory, olfactory and vertiginous), or autonomic (visceral) in type.

b) Complex (with altered consciousness): typified by 'temporal lobe epilepsy' with memory changes, déjà vu, hallucinations and automatisms. Chewing and lip-smacking movements often occur. Both types of partial seizure may be followed by loss of consciousness (secondary generalization).

Clinical tests

- *EEG* (Fig. 93): resting and sleep records may reveal and localize epileptiform discharges.
- A number of *blood tests* to exclude metabolic causes, e.g. hyper and hypocalcaemia. Remember, hypoglycaemia can present with seizures.

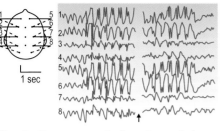

Fig. 92 Three-per-second spike and wave discharges typical of petit mal epilepsy.

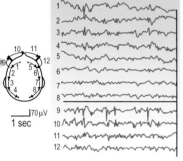

Fig. 93 Interictal EEG record in temporal lobe epilepsy showing left temporal spikes (Channels 1–4, 9, 10).

Clinical tests

- *Cranial MRI* to exclude structural brain lesions.
- *Video-EEG telemetry* allows comparison of the seizure semiology with the EEG.

Clinical examination is frequently normal, but patients treated with anti-epileptic drugs may develop drug-related unwanted effects (Fig. 94).

It is important to avoid anticonvulsant medication during pregnancy if possible, especially valproate and phenytoin which are teratogenic. Other drugs, e.g. lamotrigine and carbamazepine, are less likely to cause fetal abnormalities. If epilepsy is severe it is, of course, essential to continue medication.

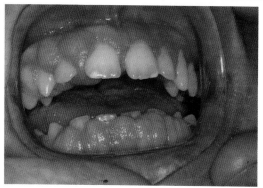

Fig. 94 Unwanted effect of phenytoin treatment: gum hyperplasia.

Aetiology

Idiopathic epilepsy: the commonest cause of epilepsy, presents in childhood or adolescence; often with a family history of epilepsy and photosensitivity on EEG.

Symptomatic epilepsy: in infants, consider congenital malformations and metabolic abnormalities; in children, consider perinatal anoxia, birth injury and neurocutaneous syndromes (Figs 95–98). In adults, consider alcohol and substance abuse, tumours and vascular and degenerative disease. In all age groups, consider trauma and infections, particularly meningitis.

Management

Patients presenting with a first seizure are often not treated with medication. For patients with recurrent seizures, treatment is based on epilepsy type (e.g. sodium valproate or lamotrigine for generalized-onset epilepsy; carbamazepine, lamotrigine or sodium valproate for partial epilepsy). Treat with monotherapy until complete control of seizures is attained or the maximal clinically tolerated dose is achieved. Advise the patient about epilepsy, about the need to stop driving and to inform DVLA, and about avoiding precipitants such as sleep deprivation and alcohol bingeing. Much idiopathic epilepsy is inherited and this is always a concern.

For intractable frequent seizures it is sometimes possible to surgically remove a discharging focus, especially from the temporal lobe. MR images may reveal focal cortical dysplasia, cavernous haemangioma (Fig. 79) or benign neoplasms as the cause of epilepsy, and surgical treatment may be very successful in such patients.

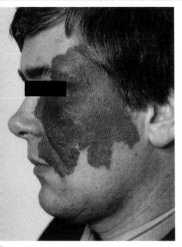

Fig. 95 Sturge–Weber naevus is often associated with epilepsy.

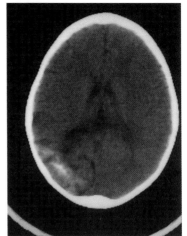

Fig. 96 CT: calcification and focal atrophy of parieto-occipital cortex in Sturge–Weber syndrome.

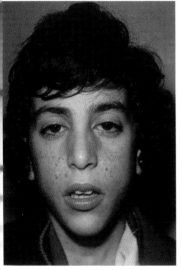

Fig. 97 Tuberous sclerosis: adenoma sebaceum.

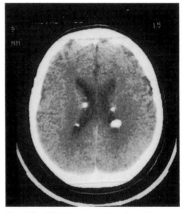

Fig. 98 CT: tuberous sclerosis with multiple periventricular calcified masses (tubers).

CNS infections

Bacterial meningitis

Aetiology

The three most common infections are:

- *Neisseria meningitidis* (meningococcus): affects young adults; may occur in epidemics.
- *Streptococcus pneumoniae* (pneumococcus): older age group; often with sinus and middle ear disease.
- *Haemophilus influenzae:* usually children younger than 6 years.

Clinical features

These include fever with headache, photophobia, neck and back stiffness, drowsiness and vomiting. Seizures may occur. Meningococcal disease causes a typical petechial rash (Fig. 99) that does not blanch with pressure, associated with fever, drowsiness and meningism. Progression of meningococcal meningitis is often very rapid—over a few hours—with either predominant meningitis or predominant septicaemia; early clinical diagnosis is *essential* and requires *alert suspicion.*

Clinical tests

If the diagnosis is clinically suspected *give antibiotics first; then investigate.* If there is papilloedema or focality to the examination, including altered consciousness, cranial CT is recommended before lumbar puncture (LP). The CSF is turbid, under increased pressure (200–300 cm), with a raised white cell count (typically 1000–10 000 per mm^3; usually 80% polymorphs), raised protein (between 1 and 5 g/L), and low glucose (<2.5 mmol/L). Gram stain may be positive (Fig. 100). Blood cultures are essential.

Management

After the initial 'blind' antibiotic regimen (usually benzyl penicillin or cefotaxime, but chloramphenicol can also be used), appropriate antibiotics (based on likely pathogens) are administered intravenously until CSF culture results are available to tailor treatment. Steroids are generally unhelpful, except in infants. In meningococcal disease, consider cefotaxime or penicillin prophylaxis for very close contacts.

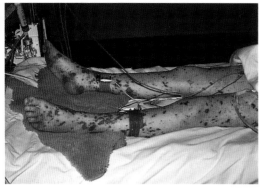

Fig. 99 Petechial rash of meningococcal septicaemia.

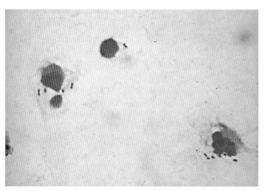

Fig. 100 CSF: Gram-positive diplococci; pneumococcal meningitis.

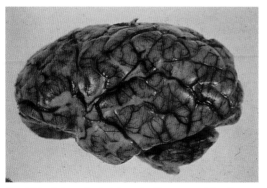

Fig. 101 Autopsy bacterial meningitis: pus overlying the cortical sulci.

Complications

These include deafness, optic atrophy, hemiplegia, cortical vein or sinus thrombosis, hydrocephalus, and subdural effusions and empyema. Autopsy shows pus in the meninges (Fig. 101). If meningitis is recurrent, consider the possibility of cranial or spinal CSF leaks, either congenital or traumatic in type, and diseases associated with immunosuppression.

Tuberculous meningitis (TBM)

There is an insidious onset with fever, headache, lethargy, anorexia, weight loss, intellectual decline and personality change. Seizures and vomiting occur in young children.

Clinical tests

Cranial CT shows basal enhancement (Fig. 102). At LP the CSF is colourless, but may be turbid, under slightly raised pressure (200–250 mm), with 50–400 white cells (mainly lymphocytes), raised protein (1–2 g/L) and either normal or low glucose level (<50% blood glucose). The differential diagnosis includes fungal and carcinomatous meningitis. Ziehl–Neelsen staining may show acid-fast bacilli (Fig. 103); PCR is a reliable technique to identify acid-fast bacilli in CSF.

Management

Treatment with antituberculous chemotherapy, e.g. isoniazid (with pyridoxine supplements), rifampicin, ethambutol and pyrazinamide. Steroids may be useful. Complications include inappropriate antidiuretic hormone (ADH) secretion, hydrocephalus and tuberculoma formation (Fig. 104).

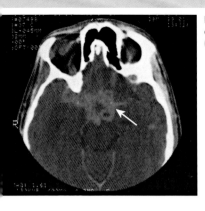

Fig. 102 CT: enhancement of basal exudate in tuberculous meningitis (arrow).

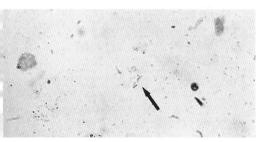

Fig. 103 CSF: acid-fast bacilli (cluster in centre) in Ziehl–Neelsen preparation (arrow).

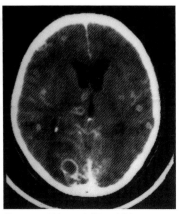

Fig. 104 Enhanced CT: multiple tuberculomas appear as solid or ring enhancing lesions.

Fungal meningitis

Aetiology

Fungal meningitis is most frequently associated with immunocompromised patients, organ transplantation, malignancy, steroid treatment or connective tissue diseases. In the UK cryptococcal infection is the most common, although *Candida*, mucormycosis and others may occur.

Clinical tests

CSF shows less than 300 white cells (usually a mix of polymorphs and lymphocytes), raised protein (although rarely more than 1.5 g/L) and normal or slightly depressed glucose level. India ink preparations may show fungal cells or hyphae (Fig. 105). Specific antibody tests and PCR tests are available.

Management

In cryptococcal infection, amphotericin B and flucytosine may be used. The mortality risk is high.

Cerebral abscess

Aetiology

Cerebral abscess can result from direct spread of infection from paranasal sinuses (frontal lobe abscess) or from middle ear and mastoid disease (temporal lobe and cerebellum). Alternatively, blood-borne infection from lung disease (abscess, pneumonia or tuberculosis, Fig. 104), endocarditis or cyanotic congenital heart disease may occur. *Subdural empyema* may also follow trauma and neurosurgery. Any organism may be involved; the most common are streptococci, staphylococci and anaerobes.

Clinical features

These include raised intracranial pressure (headache, drowsiness and vomiting), focal signs, seizures, fever and varying degrees of meningism.

Clinical tests

Cranial CT or MRI shows a mass lesion with ring enhancement (Fig. 106). Lumbar puncture is not indicated. Cranial sinus and chest radiographs, blood cultures and appropriate cultures of aspirated pus may be performed.

Management

An aggressive regimen of broad-spectrum antibiotics should be administered, with anticonvulsants and steroids as needed. Assess response regularly with serial MRI and consider surgical aspiration or excision. Prognosis is worse with multiloculated abscesses and especially if intraventricular or subarachnoid rupture occurs (Fig. 107).

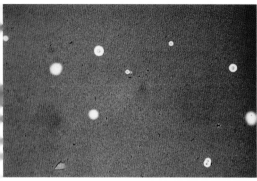

Fig. 105 CSF: cryptococcal cells outlined in an India ink preparation; specific molecular techniques are also available for diagnosis, but CSF examination can be instantly diagnostic.

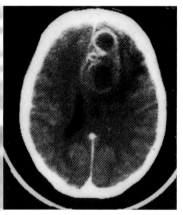

Fig. 106 Large multiloculated frontal lobe abscess showing ring enhancement and midline shift as seen on CT scan.

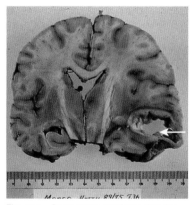

Fig. 107 Postmortem specimen showing chronic, thick-walled temporal lobe abscess that has ruptured into the subarachnoid space (arrow).

Viral meningitis

Viral meningitis is most frequently caused by one of the enteroviruses (echovirus/Coxsackie).

Clinical features

An acute illness with headache, photophobia, malaise, and neck stiffness, often preceded by fever and chills. Clear CSF under increased pressure typically yields 10–1000 lymphocytes, a protein rarely greater than 1 g/L, and normal glucose concentration.

Management

No treatment is required once bacterial meningitis is excluded, and a full recovery occurs over some days.

Viral encephalitis

Herpes simplex virus (usually type 1) is a common cause of serious viral encephalitis (Fig. 108).

Clinical features

Meningeal symptoms are generally rather mild, but there is progressive depression of consciousness, with focal features, including seizures and hemiplegia. Cranial CT, often the first investigation in hospital, initially shows swelling and low density within one or both temporal lobes, not in a vascular territory, often with scattered haemorrhages. MRI reveals these changes in more detail. Later there is focal atrophy (Fig. 109). The CSF is often under greatly increased pressure and contains up to 1000 lymphocytes, with a normal or sometimes slightly reduced glucose and increased protein concentration (1–1.5 g/L). The EEG may show background slowing and may reveal characteristic bitemporal periodic complexes at regular 2–3 second intervals. Blood and CSF serology is occasionally rewarding. The virus is difficult to isolate from CSF but PCR is a quick and reliable diagnostic technique.

Management

Treat with i.v. aciclovir at first clinical suspicion and manage raised intracranial pressure with steroids. Anticonvulsants should be prescribed as necessary. The mortality is about 20%, even with treatment, and many survivors are left with permanent deficits, usually amnesia and seizures. Early antiviral therapy is essential.

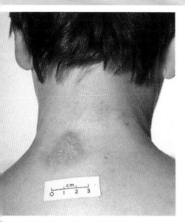

Fig. 108 Typical herpetic lesion on neck. H. simplex encephalitis, however, is usually a primary CNS infection via a nasal entry portal or on the lip, glans penis or vulva.

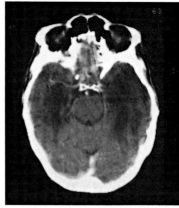

Fig. 109 Bitemporal low density in old herpes simplex encephalitis seen on CT scan.

Other viral infections

Progressive multifocal leukoencephalopathy (PML) (Fig. 110) is caused by JC virus, a papovavirus; it occurs mainly in immunocompromised subjects, especially in HIV/AIDS.

Neoplastic meningitis

Malignant invasion of the meninges with carcinoma, lymphoma or sarcoma can lead to a meningitic syndrome with a raised CSF protein, low glucose and with neoplastic and inflammatory cells in the CSF. Cranial nerve palsies are common with hydrocephalus and fever. The prognosis is very poor and chemotherapy not very effective.

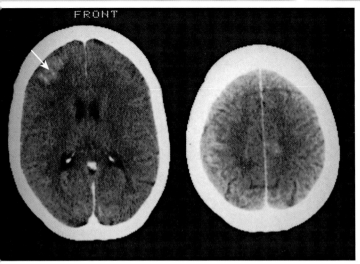

Fig. 110 Progressive multifocal leukoencephalopathy (PML) seen on CT scan. Diffuse low-density change in white matter with small haemorrhage in the right frontal area (arrow). PML may complicate HIV/AIDS. See also Fig. 192.

23 Multiple sclerosis

Multiple sclerosis

Multiple sclerosis (MS) is a demyelinating disease characterized by neurological symptoms and signs indicative of two or more lesions disseminated within the central nervous system (CNS), both in time and space. These classical clinical criteria have been codified in terms of MRI features of high specificity and good sensitivity:

- One or more T2 bright lesions in two or more of four characteristic locations: periventricular, juxtacortical, infratentorial or spinal.
- One or more T2 bright lesions at any follow-up MRI study.

Prevalence

MS is commoner in women (ratio 1.8:1.0). It begins at age 10–60 years, but most often in the third and fourth decades.

Aetiology

The cause is unknown, but demyelination appears to occur from cytokine release as a 'bystander effect' from an immune-based disorder of small blood vessels in the brain. There is an increasing risk with increasing latitude. There is a familial predisposition. An association with HLA-DR2 exists.

Clinical features

Typical presentations include optic neuritis (Fig. 111), brainstem features (vertigo, diplopia, nystagmus and ataxia) and spastic paraparesis with sphincter disturbance and impotence. Suggestive features include trigeminal neuralgia, facial myokymia, L'hermitte's sign (electric tingling in limbs and spine on neck flexion) and Uthoff's phenomena (fatigue and exacerbation of symptoms with heat or exercise). The course is either relapsing and remitting (RRMS) (Fig. 54), often with a phase of secondary progression (SPMS), or primary progressive (PPMS) (Fig. 53), particularly if older than age 40 years.

There is no specific diagnostic test; the diagnosis is clinical, and dependent on MRI criteria. MRI often shows multiple lesions, typically in a periventricular location (Figs 112 and 113) and within the brainstem and cerebellum. Acute demyelinating lesions enhance after contrast.

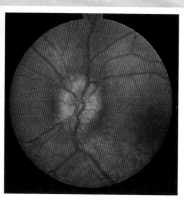

Fig. 111 Optic disc swelling in acute optic neuritis; this is always accompanied by a central field defect, although this may be minor.

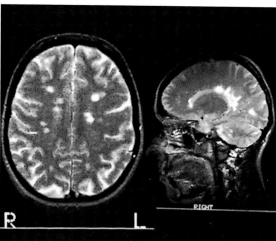

Fig. 112 Brain MRI. T2 image. High signal periventricular lesions in MS.

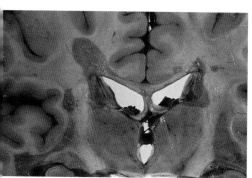

Fig. 113 Postmortem specimen showing multiple white matter plaques.

Clinical features	CSF examination reveals oligoclonal bands on isoelectric focusing (Fig. 114) and in active MS may sometimes show up to 50 mononuclear cells. The total protein may be slightly increased, although rarely above 1 g/L; the glucose level is normal. Visual evoked responses may be delayed, revealing evidence of a subclinical lesion in the optic nerve (Fig. 115). The characteristic pathological lesion seen in acute MS is perivascular cuffing with mononuclear cells and lymphocytes (Fig. 116).
Management	Newly introduced treatments promise effective suppression of the immune-based inflammation leading to demyelination, and modify the clinical course. Beta-interferon therapy reduces the risk of relapses in relapsing-remitting MS and lessens the risk of disability. New anticytokine medications are promising. Specific antispastic medications are moderately effective. Urinary dysfunction is troublesome but may respond to atropine-like drugs. Short courses of high-dose steroids shorten exacerbations. Physiotherapy can be very helpful if used appropriately after a relapse.

Other demyelinating diseases

These are rare. They include acute disseminated encephalomyelitis (ADEM)—a self-limited disorder, central pontine myelinolysis and Marchiafava–Bignami disease, and X-linked adrenomyeloleukodystrophy. Devic's disease (neuromyelitis optica) in which optic neuritis is associated with an inflammatory myelopathy is due to antibodies to the aquaporin receptor.

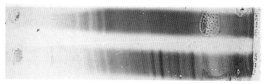

Fig. 114 CSF isoelectric focusing; normal (above) and MS patient (below). Oligoclonal bands (dark vertical lines on bottom trace) of IgG are seen.

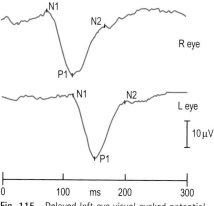

Fig. 115 Delayed left eye visual evoked potential (P1).

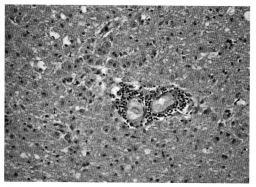

Fig. 116 Mononuclear cell perivascular cuffing in acute MS.

24 Involuntary movement disorders

Clinical features

Idiopathic Parkinson's disease

The four classic features are bradykinesia, rest tremor at 4–6 Hz, rigidity and impaired postural reflexes. Passive rotation of the wrist or elbow reveals cogwheel-like rigidity. Bradykinesia is especially disabling, causing delay in initiation of movement, which is itself slow. Fine movements such as writing (Fig. 117) become increasingly difficult. Walking is slowed, with small steps (shuffling gait), difficulty in turning and failure to swing the arms. The posture is flexed, with the head and back bowed, and the arms held partially flexed (Fig. 118). The face is immobile—the 'parkinsonian mask'. Instability and falling become problems. Autonomic features and dementia may develop late in the disease course. The sense of smell is often impaired.

Parkinson's disease is a common movement disorder, especially in older people. The main pathological abnormality is neuronal loss in the substantia nigra pars compacta (Figs 119 and 120). This leads to depletion of dopamine in the corpus striatum (Fig. 121). Surviving nigral neurons show a characteristic inclusion, the Lewy body (Fig. 122). In addition to idiopathic Parkinson's disease, parkinsonian features result from neuroleptic drug toxicity and as a presumed autoimmune disorder, encephalitis lethargica (perhaps induced by viral infection). The toxic drug 1-methyl-4-phenyl-1, 2, 5, 6-tetrahydropyridine (MTPT), a pethidine analogue, produces profound acute parkinsonism. Manganese toxicity can also cause a parkinsonian syndrome, but no common environmental cause is recognized. Parkinsonism is often inherited (various mutations are known) and a genetic component may underlie many sporadic cases.

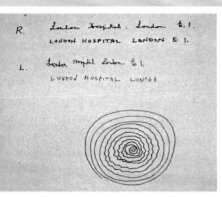

Fig. 117 The handwriting of a patient with Parkinson's disease. Micrographia and a tremulous spiral.

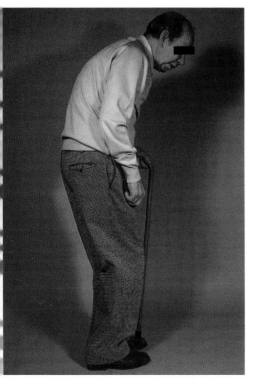

Fig. 118 Parkinson's disease, showing rigid, flexed posture at an advanced stage (off treatment).

Management

The essential of treatment is to provide an external source of dopamine (L-dopa is a precursor of dopamine) or a dopaminergic analogue. Dopamine replacement using L-dopa combined with a peripheral dopa decarboxylase inhibitor provides remarkable symptomatic relief in the idiopathic disease, although less so in atypical syndromes. After about 5 years' treatment, 50% of patients with idiopathic Parkinson's disease develop motor fluctuations, called the *on-off phenomenon*. Commonly, the duration of action of L-dopa becomes progressively shorter (*wearing-off effect*), and there may be sudden swings between profound immobility and dyskinesia (*motor fluctuations*). Other therapeutic options include dopaminergic drugs (e.g. pergolide), which are often used from the onset of therapy, and selegiline, which provides slight symptomatic relief and may slow disease progression. Anticholinergic medications are still sometimes used, especially for tremor, which responds less well to L-dopa. Stereotactic lesioning of the pallidum for tremor has been largely replaced by subthalamic stimulation, which can relieve both tremor and bradykinesia in intractable cases.

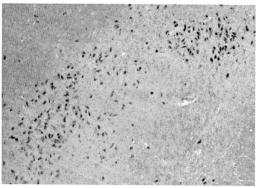

Fig. 119 Normal substantia nigra. Note normal complement of pigmented dopamine cells.

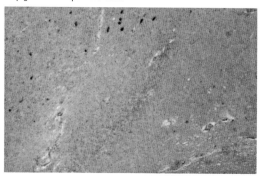

Fig. 120 Parkinsonian substantia nigra shows marked absence of pigmented cells.

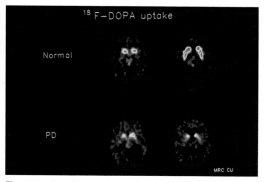

Fig. 121 A positron-emission tomography (PET) scan showing reduced 18F-dopa uptake in the basal ganglia in Parkinson's disease (PD) compared with a normal subject. Most patients with idiopathic PD show this abnormality.

Parkinson plus syndromes

A small proportion of patients who present with parkinsonian symptoms have atypical features and suffer from a 'Parkinson plus syndrome':

Progressive supranuclear palsy: recognized by a prominent vertical supranuclear gaze palsy (downward movements affected before upward), with axial rigidity, loss of balance and stance, and progressive dementia.

Multiple system atrophy: shows major early autonomic disturbance (incontinence, postural hypotension) with combinations of pyramidal (brisk reflexes, extensor plantar responses), cerebellar (dysarthria, ataxia) and parkinsonian features, especially rigidity.

Neuroleptic drugs: can lead to atypical parkinsonism, often with pronounced dystonia and with tremor, after prolonged exposure, e.g. in the management of major psychoses.

Essential tremor

There is a fast irregular tremor, often worse on action and on postural maintenance, and not present at rest, involving upper more than lower limbs, and often affecting face, lips and head. It may be familial. The cardinal features of parkinsonism are absent. Propranolol may be helpful. In most cases the tremor commences after middle age.

Other basal ganglia disorders

Disease of the basal ganglia can lead to a variety of different movement abnormalities, such as chorea, athetosis, dystonia (Fig. 123) and ballismus—a kinetic 'throwing' movement of a limb. Very similar involuntary movements may occur with a number of different causes. Wilson's disease, a defect of copper metabolism, must always be excluded; it is fatal unless treated.

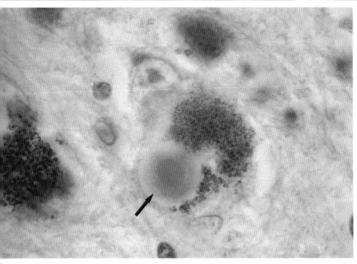

Fig. 122 Lewy body. High-power photomicrographs of the Lewy body—acytoplasmic eosinophilic inclusion body with a clear surrounding halo. Lewy bodies contain alpha-synuclein.

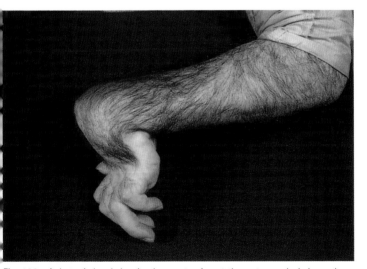

Fig. 123 A dystonic hand showing hyperextension at the metacarpal-phalangeal joints and flexion at the wrist.

Huntington's disease

This is a chronic degenerative disorder, particularly involving the caudate nuclei and cortex, giving rise to chorea and dementia. It is inherited in an autosomal dominant pattern (chromosome 6). The DNA abnormality consists of a sequence of trinucleotide repeats, larger numbers of repeats being associated with earlier onset disease.

Clinical features

Choreiform movements, evident in face and limbs (Fig. 124), and progressive dementia, with onset usually in the fourth or fifth decade, dominate the clinical picture. Initially, the chorea may be very mild but it progresses with time. Since the mutation rate is low, a family history is almost always known or discoverable. The clinical diagnosis can be confirmed by DNA testing, and preclinical diagnosis is possible in affected families, a test with major ethical and personal implications. There is a high risk of suicide.

Treatment is symptomatic. Reserpine-like drugs, e.g. tetrabenazine, that deplete basal ganglia dopamine, confer moderate benefit on the involuntary movements but do not modify the underlying disease or the dementia.

Other causes of chorea include Sydenham's chorea, associated with post-streptococcal antibodies to basal ganglia neurons, and rheumatic fever. Chorea may also occur in SLE and after pregnancy.

Athetosis

This is characterized by slow writhing postures of the limbs. It is mainly seen as a form of congenital cerebral palsy associated with anoxia or kernicterus or, in adults, after cerebral trauma.

Dystonia

Dystonia is a movement disorder in which there are sustained muscle contractions, frequently causing twisting and repetitive movements and abnormal postures (Fig. 123). It may be localized or generalized.

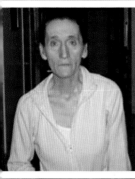

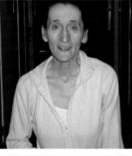

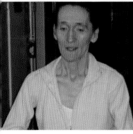

Fig. 124 Chorea in Huntington's disease. Continual facial twitches and hand gestures are characteristic.

*Clinical
features*

Focal dystonia affects one part of the body; *generalized dystonia* affects the limbs and trunk more diffusely.

Adult onset *focal dystonias* are 12 times more common than generalized forms. The most common focal dystonias are blepharospasm (Fig. 125), spasmodic torticollis (Fig. 126) and occupational dystonias (movement-related dystonia) such as writer's cramp and musician's dystonia (Fig. 127). Their onset is usually between the ages of 20 and 50 years and the course is often slowly progressive.

Generalized dystonia occurs sporadically in one-third of patients and as an autosomal recessive or dominant disorder in a further third. The remainder develop dystonia secondary to other conditions, including cerebral palsy and use of neuroleptic drugs. It may also occur in Wilson's disease. In *torsion dystonia*, the onset is usually localized, starting before the age of 11 years, and gradually becomes widespread.

In general, treatment of these involuntary movement disorders is unsatisfactory. Acute drug-induced dyskinesias should be treated with an intravenous anticholinergic agent. Dystonia may be helped by high-dose anticholinergics, and sometimes by L-dopa. Blepharospasm and spasmodic torticollis are treated symptomatically by injection of botulinum toxin into the orbicularis oculi and neck muscles, respectively.

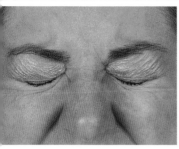

Fig. 125 Blepharospasm.

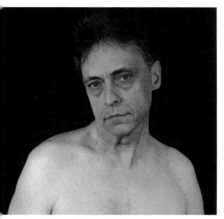

Fig. 126 Spasmodic torticollis.

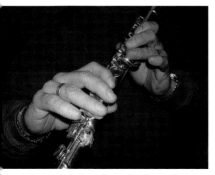

Fig. 127 Musician's dystonia. The flautist's left little finger has tonically detached itself from the key, making it difficult to continue playing.

Polyneuropathies are disorders of the peripheral nervous system as a whole, due to genetic, e.g. Charcot–Marie–Tooth disease (CMT), or acquired disorders (e.g. Guillain–Barré syndrome or diabetic neuropathy). In mononeuropathies, individual peripheral nerves or nerve roots are affected by local processes such as pressure, entrapment, trauma or inflammation.

Polyneuropathies

Clinical features

Polyneuropathies cause symmetrical distal sensory loss and weakness. Distal motor signs, e.g. wasting and weakness of the feet and legs (Fig. 128), are prominent in axonal neuropathies. In demyelinating neuropathies, such as Guillain–Barré syndrome (Fig. 129), there is diffuse, proximally predominant weakness, with preserved muscle bulk and prominent dysaesthesiae or pain.

In some inherited progressive neuropathies, e.g. Refsum's disease and CMT, there is maldevelopment of the distal parts of the limbs, especially the toes, e.g. pes cavus (Fig. 130). In chronic demyelinating neuropathies and leprosy (Hansen's disease), there is hypertrophy of the cutaneous nerves (Fig. 131).

In long-standing peripheral neuropathies associated with severe distal sensory loss, there is trophic damage to tendons and joints, leading to progressive deformity of the joints of the feet, ankles and knees, including Charcot joint deformities (Fig. 132).

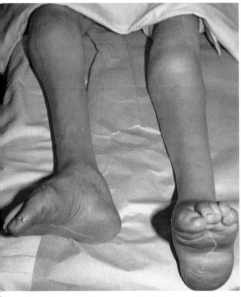

Fig. 128 Distal wasting and weakness in an axonal neuropathy.

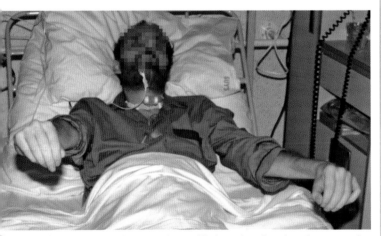

Fig. 129 Guillain–Barré syndrome; weakness of limbs and trunk, and respiratory muscles requiring ITU therapy.

Investigations

Look for signs of systemic disease, e.g. diabetes mellitus, cancer, vasculitis, dysproteinaemia and leprosy. Is there a family history? Is the neuropathy acute? Is there symmetrical polyneuropathy, mononeuropathy or multiple involvement of single nerves? Is there biochemical or imaging evidence of systemic disease? Is the motor or sensory nerve conduction velocity slowed (<35 m/s) as in *demyelinating neuropathy*, or is it more or less normal, as in *axonal neuropathy*? Is there conduction block, i.e. lower amplitude muscle action potential recorded from a distal muscle after proximal stimulation than after distal stimulation of the same nerve? This is a sign of dysimmune demyelinating neuropathy, especially Guillain–Barré disease and multifocal motor neuropathy with conduction block (MMN). CSF examination may be helpful, showing a raised protein in demyelinating neuropathies, and malignant cells in neoplastic infiltration. Specific antibody tests, e.g. antiGM$_1$ antibodies and antigliadin antibodies, may reveal causation.

Nerve biopsy

Sural nerve biopsy near the ankle is occasionally useful, particularly if vasculitis is suspected. However, quantitative neurophysiological tests, genetic tests and specific antibody studies have rendered diagnostic biopsy largely redundant.

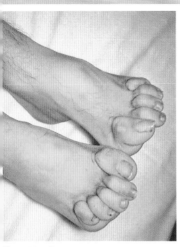

Fig. 130 Pes cavus.

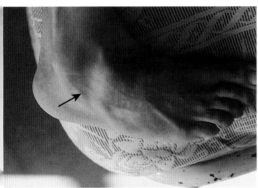

Fig. 131 Hypertrophy of the distal cutaneous branch of the sural nerve on the lateral border of the foot in HNSM type 1, a genetically-determined demyelinating neuropathy.

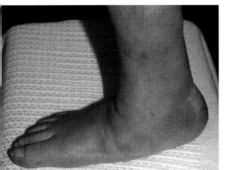

Fig. 132 Weakness of the arch of the foot in Charcot–Marie–Tooth disease (HMSN).

Clinical types

Guillain–Barré syndrome

This is a common, acute, inflammatory demyelinating polyneuropathy that follows a minor acute infection. There is distal and/or proximal weakness, often affecting the face (Fig. 133). Respiratory muscle involvement is frequent and potentially fatal; assess ventilatory capacity at least daily in the acute active phase. There may be slight distal sensory loss and tendon reflexes are absent. In general, the prognosis is excellent: treatment with i.v. gamma globulin at presentation will accelerate recovery. A relapsing, chronic form, chronic inflammatory demyelinating polyradiculoneuropathy (CIDP), is steroid responsive. Cases following *C. jejuni* infection are especially severe and often primarily axonal.

Other polyneuropathies

Charcot–Marie–Tooth disease (HMSN):   a group of hereditary neuropathies of several different clinical types and genetic loci. The type 1 disorder is demyelinating and the type 2 axonal in type. There is a symmetrical sensorimotor neuropathy with pes cavus. Hereditary liability to pressure palsies is a disorder related to type 1 HMSN due to a point mutation or deletion at the same genetic locus.

Paraproteinemic neuropathy: a sensorimotor neuropathy with slowed conduction velocity, occurs with monoclonal gamma and M-band proteins, in the elderly and in association with lymphomas or plasma cell dyscrasia.

Paraneoplastic neuropathies: sensorimotor neuropathy may complicate cancer or be the primary presentation of occult cancers, especially lymphomas.

Hansen's disease (leprosy):   a generalized neuropathy due to mycobacterial infection, often causing *multiple single nerve palsies* and a characteristic 'leonine facies' with coarsened features. Small zones of *anaesthetic* depigmented skin, sometimes with a raised red margin occur especially on relatively cold parts of the body, e.g. the face. The peripheral nerves are enlarged and nodular. Hypoaesthetic, depigmented skin lesions and nodular enlargement of peripheral nerves, especially cutaneous nerves, occur.

Hereditary amyloid neuropathies: amyloid is deposited in peripheral nerves (Fig. 134), causing hypertrophied nerves with damage to the myelin of affected nerve fibres and therefore slowed nerve conduction velocity.

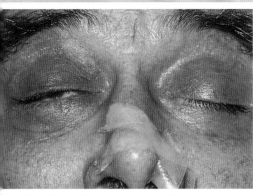

Fig. 133 Bilateral facial weakness in Guillain–Barré neuropathy.

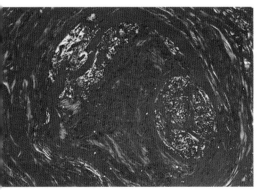

Fig. 134 Apple-green fluorescence of amyloid deposition seen in a nerve biopsy stained with Congo red.

Mononeuropathies

Aetiology

The median, ulnar, radial and common peroneal nerves, as well as the lateral cutaneous nerve of the thigh, are commonly damaged by external pressure, by direct injury or by entrapment in interosseous and intramuscular canals.

Clinical syndromes

Median nerve palsy: (Fig. 135) caused by entrapment in the carpal tunnel on the flexor aspect of the wrist. The nerve is trapped and compressed at this site, resulting in weakness and wasting of the thenar eminence, with sensory disturbance in the median-innervated skin of the palm of the hand. There is often pain in the forearm, especially at night. Nerve conduction studies show slowed nerve conduction velocity, with conduction block, across the carpal tunnel.

Ulnar nerve palsy: atrophy and weakness of intrinsic hand muscles (Fig. 136), with sensory loss on the inner border of the hand, both palmar and dorsal. There is weakness of all intrinsic hand muscles, with a posture of interphalangeal flexion and metacarpophalangeal extension affecting the medial two digits (Figs 136 and 137). The nerve is damaged by pressure/entrapment at the elbow (in or just below the olecranon groove) and there is tenderness at this site, with pain and tingling referred into the distribution of the nerve in the hand (Tinel's sign).

Radial nerve palsy: the classic 'Saturday night palsy', usually due to pressure injury in the spiral groove of the humerus or fracture of the humerus. It presents with wrist and finger drop. There is a small area of sensory loss in the anatomical snuffbox.

Common peroneal nerve palsy: presents with weakness of ankle dorsiflexion and eversion, and sensory impairment on the lateral aspect of the foot and leg. The ankle jerk is normal (see page 35).

Meralgia paraesthetica: consists of an unpleasant patch of irritable numbness on the lateral thigh due to compression of the lateral cutaneous nerve of the thigh beneath the inguinal ligament, especially in obese people, or following surgery with the legs elevated in the 'stirrup' position.

Diabetic amyotrophy: an acute painful proximal lower limb motor neuropathy occurs in the context of poor diabetic control, or at diagnosis. Recovery is slow.

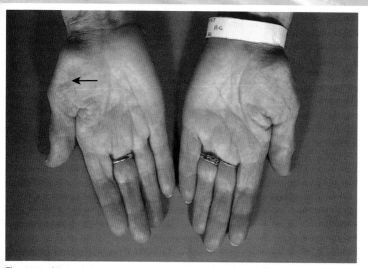

Fig. 135 Bilateral thenar wasting in carpal tunnel syndrome. The hypothenar eminence is normal.

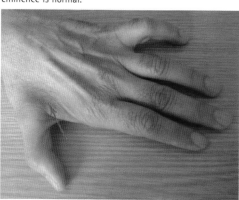

Fig. 136 Ulnar nerve palsy; wasted first dorsal interosseus and lumbricals with flexed abducted digit 5.

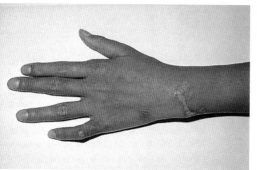

Fig. 137 Ulnar nerve palsy, with typical D4 and D5 finger posture.

Duchenne muscular dystrophy (DMD)

This X-linked myopathy is a disabling, progressive and fatal, sex-linked recessive, inherited disorder, affecting 1 in 3500 male births. The disorder progresses from difficulty walking and climbing at age 3–5 years to total dependency by about the age of 12 years and death around the age of 20 years. Most DMD boys never run.

Aetiology

In DMD there is absence of dystrophin, a cytoskeletal protein constituent of the framework of the muscle cell membrane. The dystrophin gene is located on the short arm of the X chromosome at the Xp21 position, the site of large DNA deletions responsible for most cases of the disease. Abnormalities of this gene can be recognized in white blood cells. *Becker's muscular dystrophy* is a less severe form of the Xp21 disorder, due to point deletions or mutations, presenting in older boys and with a slower progression.

Clinical features

Cardiac involvement is frequent, especially in the Becker variant, but the external ocular, pelvic sphincter and distal hand muscles tend to be spared. Proximal weakness leads to Gower's manoeuvre in standing from sitting on the floor (Fig. 138). Affected limb muscles, especially calves and deltoids, usually show hypertrophy from fibrosis and fatty infiltration in the earlier stages (Fig. 139). Joint contractures and respiratory difficulties develop.

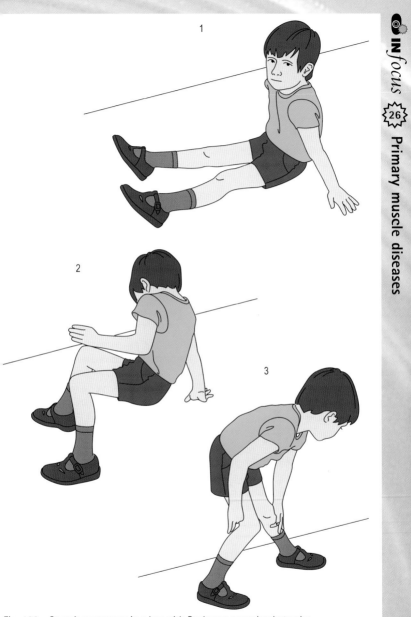

Fig. 138 Gower's manoeuvre in a boy with Duchenne muscular dystrophy.

Investigations

The blood creatine kinase (CK) level is markedly raised. The *muscle biopsy* (Fig. 140) shows increased thickness of interfascicular and endomysial fibrous connective tissue (blue-green in illustration), large rounded, densely stained 'hyaline' fibres and smaller rounded fibres, with foci of degeneration and regeneration of individual fibres.

EMG and muscle biopsy are useful studies in patients with myopathy of unclear cause. Imaging of muscle can clearly delineate the pattern of muscle involvement (Fig. 141).

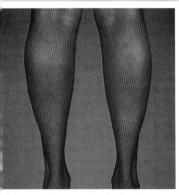

Fig. 139 Hypertrophy of calves in Duchenne muscular dystrophy.

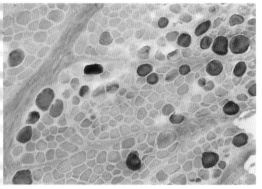

Fig. 140 Muscle biopsy in Duchenne dystrophy.

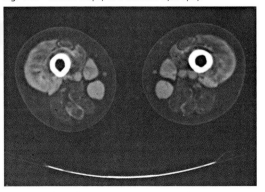

Fig. 141 MRI thigh muscles. Involvement of thigh muscles in limb-girdle muscular dystrophy (LGMD). The low attenuation muscles are severely involved.

Facioscapulohumeral muscular dystrophy (FSH)

This is an uncommon, autosomal dominant, inherited disease that is a specific clinical syndrome with a recognized causative mutation on the telomere of Ch4q.

Weakness particularly affects facial, periscapular and biceps brachii muscles with similar involvement of thigh and pelvic girdle muscles in the later stages of the disease (Fig. 142). The heart is not involved, but respiratory muscles become weak later, and life expectancy is decreased.

Oculopharyngeal muscular dystrophy

This condition involves ocular and pharyngeal muscles (Fig. 143) as a dominantly inherited disorder of late onset. There is mild proximal muscle weakness.

Progressive ocular myopathy

Most cases have a primary mitochondrial causation, inherited through mitochondrial DNA mutations. There may be associated cerebellar ataxia, deafness, macular degeneration, peripheral neuropathy and metabolic myopathy.

Scapuloperoneal muscular dystrophy

Periscapular muscles are relatively selectively affected in scapuloperoneal muscular dystrophy (Fig. 144). Weakness of the periscapular muscles makes the shoulders unstable because of the inability to fix the position of the scapulae against a load.

Limb–girdle muscular dystrophies

In this group of syndromes, proximal or distal weakness develops in childhood, adolescence or adult life. Some are associated with life-threatening cardiomyopathy. Autosomal dominant or recessive syndromes are recognized. There may be involvement of the brain in some, and others show distinctive clinical and histological features, e.g. rigid spine syndrome. In most, DNA mutations are known and testable for diagnosis.

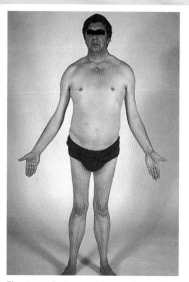

Fig. 142 Facioscapulohumeral muscular dystrophy, showing atrophy of proximal and upper arm muscles, with lordosis and facial involvement.

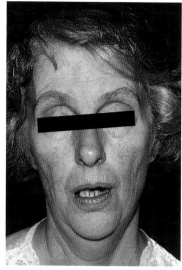

Fig. 143 Oculopharyngeal muscular dystrophy, with ptosis, weakness of extraocular muscles and facial and bulbar muscular weakness.

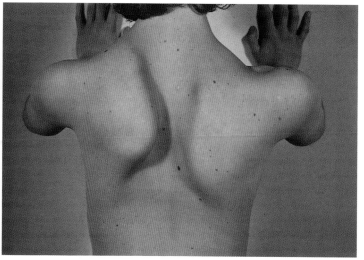

Fig. 144 Periscapular muscle weakness causes winging of the scapulae.

Myotonic dystrophy

This is a dominantly inherited disorder. Proximal myotonic myopathy (PROMM) is a milder phenotype with a different causative mutation.

Myotonia is a persistent discharge of muscle fibres after cessation of voluntary contraction or after a mechanical stimulus, due to ion channel dysfunction at the muscle membrane ('channelopathy'). There is therefore delayed relaxation after contraction. In *myotonic dystrophy*, there is generalized myotonia with ptosis and weakness of the face, the distal limb muscles and the sternomastoids. This produces a characteristic facial and body appearance, with a wasted neck and face (Figs 145 and 146). Cardiomyopathy with arrhythmias, oesophageal dysfunction, constipation, mild glucose intolerance and testicular atrophy may occur. In other *congenital myotonic syndromes*, e.g. cold-induced myotonia and potassium-related myotonia, dystrophic features are absent.

Investigations

The EMG is diagnostic; myotonic discharges produce a 'dive-bomber' or 'revving motor bike' sound of varying frequency and amplitude that can be recorded as a series of spike discharges (Fig. 147). The mutation on chromosome 19 consists of a sequence of trinucleotide repeats, accounting for the variable age of onset and severity of the disorder.

Inflammatory myopathies

Dermatomyositis and polymyositis

Inflammatory myopathies are characterized by autoimmune-mediated muscle fibre necrosis. Dermatomyositis is usually acute; in adults (usually older than 50 years) it may sometimes be a remote manifestation of cancer. The childhood variety of the disease has a marked vascular component. Polymyositis also occurs as a component of mixed connective tissue disease. There is muscle tenderness, weakness and, in dermatomyositis, a violaceous rash, especially in areas exposed to light (Fig. 148). The erythrocyte sedimentation rate (ESR) and CK are raised, and the EMG and muscle biopsy are diagnostic (Fig. 149).

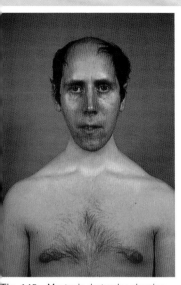

Fig. 145 Myotonic dystrophy, showing frontal baldness and characteristic facial appearance.

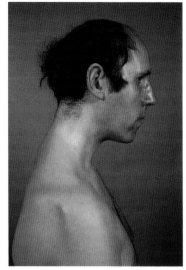

Fig. 146 Weakness of sternomastoids and neck extensors is a feature of myotonic dystrophy.

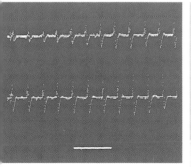

Fig. 147 Myotonic discharges on an EMG, showing the incremental amplitude and gradually changing frequency of the discharge from a single muscle fibre. Bar: 20 ms.

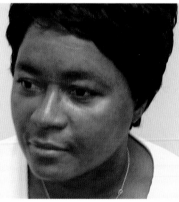

Fig. 148 Dermatomyositis. There is a subtle rash on the face and forehead.

Metabolic myopathies

These include glycogen storage diseases, disorders of lipid metabolism and mitochondrial myopathies. They are inherited disorders of metabolism, often but not necessarily restricted to muscle, usually due to single enzyme deficiencies. Most cause severe childhood onset syndromes or milder adult onset syndromes.

Acid maltase deficiency in adults presents as a late-onset progressive myopathy, causing weakness, fatigue and diaphragmatic paralysis leading to sleep apnoea. The vacuolar appearance of the muscle biopsy (Fig. 150) is due to accumulation of glycogen within lysosomes. In childhood this enzyme defect causes myopathy, cardiomyopathy, hepatosplenomegaly and mental retardation.

In *mitochondrial myopathies*, fatigue, lactic acidosis and CNS features, including ophthalmoplegia, are the main features. In muscle biopsies there are accumulations of abnormal enlarged mitochondria at the edges of type 1 muscle fibres, shown in the NADH reaction (Fig. 151). Renal tubular acidosis and CNS involvement occur in some cases. The mitochondrial myoencephalopathies are also maternally inherited and due to defects in mitochondrial DNA.

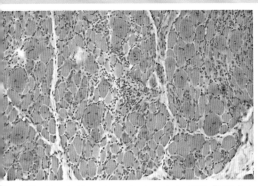

Fig. 149 Muscle biopsy in acute dermatomyositis. There is a diffuse inflammatory cell response, with muscle fibre necrosis and regeneration.

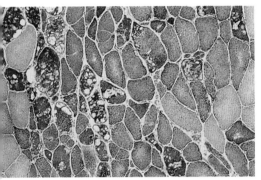

Fig. 150 Acid maltase deficiency (adult onset type). There is a prominent vacuolar myopathy.

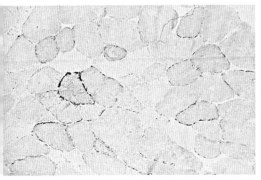

Fig. 151 Mitochondrial myopathy showing accumulation of mitochondria at the edges of type 1 muscle fibres as succinic dehydrogenase-positive structures.

27 Myasthenia gravis and related syndromes

Myasthenia gravis is an autoimmune disease in which an IgG antibody is directed against a component of the acetylcholine receptor (AChR) antigen complex at the postsynaptic part of the neuromuscular junction. These receptors are nicotinic cholinergic receptors. There is an association with autoimmune thyroid disease.

Several other antibody targets at the motor end plate are recognized, e.g. MUSK antibody myasthenia, which often affects facial muscles, and the Lambert–Eaton myasthenic syndrome (LEMS), which spares external ocular muscles but causes a myasthenic syndrome in which effort results in initial weakness followed by improvement in strength, together with autonomic features, e.g. reduced sweating, and reduced reflexes. LEMS occurs spontaneously and as a non-metastatic complication of small cell-type bronchogenic carcinoma.

Clinical features

There is fluctuating fatigability and weakness, worse at the end of the day and relieved by rest. Ptosis (Fig. 152) and weakness of external ocular muscles (Fig. 153) are common; diplopia is the presenting feature in 40% of cases. The ocular muscles often show predominant bilateral lateral rectus weakness (Fig. 154). Distal hand muscles are next most commonly affected. The disease reaches its maximal severity about a year after the onset. Weakness worsens with repeated movement or in a maintained posture (fatigability). There is no sensory loss and the tendon reflexes are normal.

Investigations

The response to test doses of anticholinesterase drugs (e.g. neostigmine) is both dramatic and diagnostic (Fig. 154). Electrodiagnostic tests reveal a decrement in the amplitude of the muscle action potential evoked by repetitive supramaximal electrical stimuli to the nerve supplying the muscle tested (Fig. 155). In health, the fourth potential of a sequence elicited at 2–30 Hz should not be more than 10% smaller than the first. Neuromuscular jitter (the variation in firing interval of individual muscle fibres innervated by a single motor unit during voluntary activation) recorded by single fibre EMG is increased.

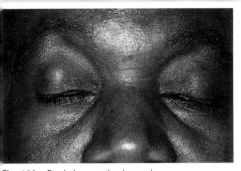

Fig. 152 Ptosis in myasthenia gravis.

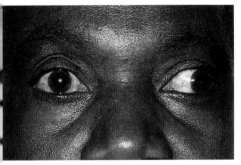

Fig. 153 Same patient as in Fig. 152 after intravenous edrophonium with improvement in ptosis to show weakness of extraocular muscles.

Management

Treatment consists of symptomatic therapy with anticholinesterase drugs and immunosuppression with azathioprine or steroids. IVIg is also used to induce remission by displacing blocking antibody in acutely ill patients.

Long-term immunosuppression with azathioprine and with daily or alternate daily steroid therapy has rendered thymectomy less used. Thymectomy induces remission, especially in the first 2 years of the disease. It has been used at the time of diagnosis in most patients, except in the very old and those with mild ocular symptoms alone. In about half of men with myasthenia and in about 10% of patients overall, there is a thymoma, a tumour of low malignancy that can usually be detected by MR scanning of the chest. In most patients, hyperplasia of the thymus is found. This thymic abnormality is thought to initiate the disturbed immune response that causes the defect in neuromuscular transmission.

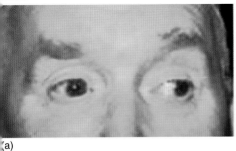

(a)

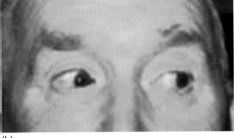

(b)

Fig. 154 Myasthenia gravis. Lateral gaze with ptosis (a) before and (b) after cholinergic therapy. The response can be quite subtle.

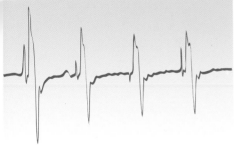

Fig. 155 Decrement in amplitude of evoked muscle action potential in 2-Hz train of stimuli to the motor nerve.

Amyotrophic lateral sclerosis (ALS)

ALS is a sporadic degenerative disorder of the lower and upper motor neurons, often with an associated fronto-temporal dementia. Its cause is unknown.

Clinical features

There is progressive weakness, usually asymmetrical at the onset, with wasting, fasciculation, spasticity and extensor plantar responses. Life expectancy is 2–3 years from diagnosis, but more rapid or slower progression is not uncommon. The peak incidence is in the sixth decade. Sensation is normal, and external ocular and sphincter muscles are not involved. The intrinsic hand muscles are often involved early (Figs 156 and 157). Widespread fasciculation occurs. Wasting and fasciculation of the tongue is particularly characteristic (Fig. 158). Cramp is common. Bulbar palsy, causing difficulty speaking and swallowing, and weakness of ventilatory muscles carry a poor prognosis. A few cases are familial, usually associated with abnormalities in the Cu–Zn superoxide dysmutase gene on chromosome 21, suggesting an excitotoxic aetiology for this form of the disease.

Investigations

The diagnosis is clinical, supported by EMG findings of widespread denervation and reinnervation, with normal motor and sensory nerve conduction studies. Imaging is important to exclude spinal cord compression. Fasciculation may be a feature of motor neuropathies, especially multifocal motor neuropathy (MMN). CSF examination is normal.

Management

Supportive care should include physiotherapy, provision of communication and mobility aids, per-enteric gastroenterostomy for feeding when swallowing becomes difficult, and elective positive pressure ventilatory assistance at night and, later, continuously if so desired. Anti-excitotoxic therapy with riluzole slightly slows progression of the disease. There is no cure. Much family support is needed.

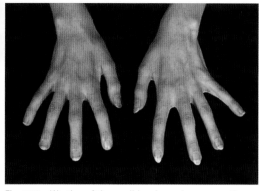

Fig. 156 Wasting of the small hand muscles seen on the dorsal aspect in motor neuron disease.

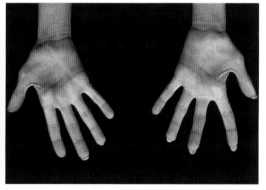

Fig. 157 View of palmar surface of hands seen in Fig. 156.

Spinal muscular atrophy (SMA)

SMA is an autosomal recessive disease, causing degeneration of anterior horn cells, without UMN involvement. An infantile form (Type 2 SMA) causes severe lifelong disability with respiratory problems and scoliosis. In Werdnig–Hoffman disease (Type 1 SMA) the child is floppy and quadriplegic from birth; death occurs by age 2 years. The common form (Type 3 SMA) is of adolescent onset, with survival for many decades. There is often rapid progression initially but then the disorder appears to become relatively stable, with rather symmetrical weakness, wasting and fasciculation. Bulbar involvement is uncommon, and ventilatory muscles are relatively spared until the end stages, when elective nocturnal ventilation may be required. These SMA syndromes are due to mutations in the *smn* gene on chromosome 13. Various other rare, late onset SMA syndromes seem to have different genetic aetiologies.

Bulbo-spinal muscular atrophy (Kennedy syndrome)

This is an X-linked disease, associated with gynaecomastia, due to mutations in the androgen receptor gene. There is bulbar and facial weakness, wasting, fasciculation and cramp, with dysphagia, and impotence. Limb-girdle muscles are moderately affected. The disease commences at any age and seems to progress slowly. Life expectancy is affected in early onset cases. Daughters of mothers with an affected son have a 50% chance of carrying the gene.

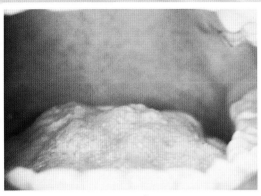

Fig. 158 Wasting of the tongue (which was also fasciculating) in ALS.

Sporadic ALS
- *Classical adult onset Charcot ALS:* about 95% of cases
- *Primary lateral sclerosis:* pure UMN syndrome, with involvement of speech and swallowing
- *Progressive bulbar palsy:* ALS beginning with bulbar and pseudobulbar palsy
- *Progressive muscular atrophy:* a pure LMN syndrome

Familial ALS syndromes (FALS)
- *SOD1 related ALS* (superoxide dismutase mutations): about 20% of all FALS, usually autosomal dominant inheritance
- *Other genetic defects* (all rare)
- *Infantile onset inherited ALS*

Neurogenic atrophy in other disorders
- *Spinal muscular atrophy:* an autosomal recessive pure LMN disorder
- *Kennedy's syndrome:* X-linked LMN syndrome of infantile, adolescent or adult onset
- *Various motor neuropathies and other disorders that may mimic ALS*

Fig. 159 Recognized types of amyotrophic lateral sclerosis.

Genetically determined degenerations may affect the cerebellum and its related pathways—sometimes called 'system degenerations'. These consist of spinocerebellar syndromes (SCA), with symmetrical ataxia of adult onset or beginning in middle life. In these disorders symmetrical cerebellar features are often associated with peripheral neuropathy, posterior column degeneration (causing profound sensory loss in the legs), autonomic features (incontinence and impotence), pigmentary retinal degeneration and deafness, and corticospinal features (causing spasticity). Dementia may also occur. Many of these clinical syndromes have been associated with specific mutations, and their classification has become more specifically based on these mutations than on their clinical features. Indeed, the phenotype of each mutation tends to be quite wide, so that even apparently discrete syndromes formerly regarded as clinically well-defined, such as Friedreich's ataxia, are now seen as syndromes with quite variable and sometimes partial manifestations associated with recognized mutations. There are thus modifier genes, as yet not well understood. The syndrome of familial spastic paraplegia (FSP) similarly is associated with a large number of specific DNA abnormalities, and with subtle variation in phenotype, but with considerable variation even within families.

Paraneoplastic cerebellar syndromes have also been recognized, associated with antibodies to Purkinje cell antigens, which have a rapidly progressive course, often with an inflammatory CSF, consisting of a lymphocytic exudate with a normal glucose. These syndromes sometimes respond to steroid therapy. They may closely mimic genetically determined cerebellar syndromes, and may be associated with paraneoplastic neuropathy and dementia.

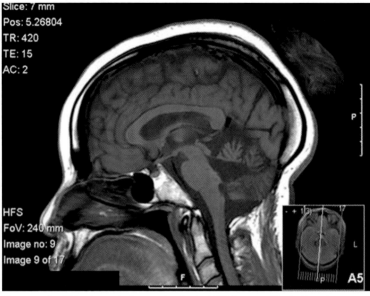

Fig. 160 Familial spinocerebellar atrophy. Sagittal MR T1 scan of brain. There is very marked atrophy of the cerebellar vermis, and of the cerebellar hemispheres, causing progressive truncal ataxia and limb ataxia.

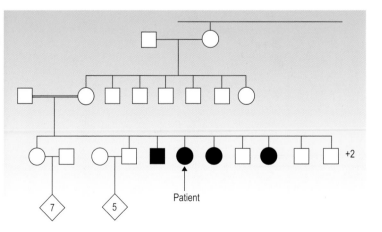

Fig. 161 Family tree showing autosomal recessive pattern of inheritance of a cerebellar degeneration (ARCA). There are several affected siblings, and the parents are therefore both carriers of the abnormal gene.

30 Spinal cord disease

Aetiology

Spinal cord disease may be degenerative, neoplastic, infective, vascular, inflammatory, developmental or traumatic.

Clinical features

Pay particular attention to the sequence of development of symptoms, and assess the motor and sensory level carefully. Intrinsic and extrinsic cord lesion cause different syndromes.

Intrinsic cord disorders cause:
- presentation with sphincter disturbance
- segmental loss of pain and temperature sensation (may not be noticed), and segmental burning dysaesthesiae from spinothalamic tract involvement
- local loss of reflexes
- segmental muscle weakness and wasting
- spastic paraparesis below level of lesion
- posterior column sensory loss below lesion level.

Intrinsic disorders are commonly inflammatory, e.g. multiple sclerosis. Intrinsic cord neoplasms, e.g. ependymoma of cauda equina and cord gliomas, are uncommon. Developmental lesions, e.g. AVM or cavernous haemangiomas, also occur, causing sudden and repeated episodes of intrinsic cord disorder. Intrinsic haematomas are uncommon but may occur with bleeding diathesis, AVM or trauma. In syringomyelia (Fig. 162) there is a cavity in the spinal cord, usually at a high cervical level, causing a characteristic clinical syndrome. It is often associated with Chiari 1 malformation in which there is herniation of the cerebellar tonsils into the foramen magnum, sometimes with hydrocephalus. Viral infection may be specific to various cell systems, e.g. herpes simplex affects sensory ganglion cells and poliomyelitis involved lower motor neurons. Vitamin B_{12} deficiency leads to a specific syndrome of combined degeneration of posterior columns and corticospinal tracts.

Extrinsic cord disorders cause:
- radicular features (root pain and segmental motor and sensory loss) at the level of the lesion
- spastic paraparesis (often asymmetric or of Brown-Séquard type)
- sensory level to pin prick and touch below lesion
- late sphincter disturbance, usually when paraparesis is severe.

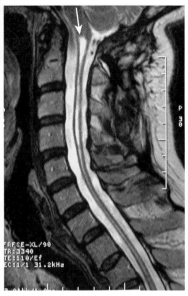

Fig. 162 MRI T2 image: syringomyelia. The spinal cord contains a fluid-filled cavity from the C1 level to the thoracic region. The cerebellar tonsils (arrow) are positioned abnormally low in the foramen magnum (Chiari 1 malformation).

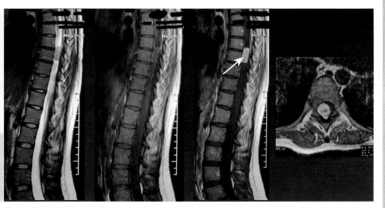

Fig. 163 MRI of neurofibroma compressing thoracic cord, presenting with paraparesis and posterior column sensory symptoms (arrow). The cord is displaced and compressed by the tumour.

Clinical features

Extrinsic syndromes occur with tumours compressing the cord, e.g. neurofibromas (Fig. 163) arising from nerve roots, meningioma or metastatic disease. Thoracic or cervical disc protrusion can also cause acute or chronic cord compression (Fig. 164). Spinal vertebral metastases, especially from lung cancer and breast cancer, cause local pain and rapidly progressive paraplegia (Fig. 165). The cord is damaged by the compression and by interference with its blood supply. Both root pain and local bony pain are frequent in malignant vertebral disease.

Cervical spondylosis with cord compression, often associated with a congenitally narrow canal, is a relatively common cause of cord compression. There is gradual onset and progression of an extrinsic syndrome, beginning with root pain and progressing to cord involvement, with a predominant spastic paraplegia. Neurosurgical decompression is necessary if the disorder is progressive and there are no adverse features, such as extreme age.

Degenerative cord disease

There are specific clinical patterns in different syndromes, with a combination of spastic paraplegia, motor neuronal syndromes (as in SMA) and autonomic dysfunction (progressive autonomic failure) and posterior column features (Friedreich's ataxia). These features are often combined with signs of cerebellar dysfunction and of basal ganglia disease, as in the *spinocerebellar degenerations (SCA syndromes)*. These can often be recognized by specific genetic tests. Posterior column degeneration may result from vitamin B_{12} deficiency, as well as from copper deficiency after gastrectomy, in chronic hepatic disease and as a paraneoplastic disorder, especially with small cell cancer of the lung.

Clinical tests

MR or CT imaging (Figs 163 and 164) are the investigations of choice, revealing cord compression, often with localized signal hyperintensity in T2 images of the cord. Intrinsic disorders, such as multiple sclerosis, will be demonstrated. Tests for B_{12} deficiency are often useful. CT scans of bony lesions (Fig. 165) are often informative. Whole-body isotope bone scanning will reveal multiple metastases. A straight X-ray at the clinical level in the spine can be a useful and cost-effective primary investigation. CSF can be studied in suspected demyelination (monoclonal IgG is present in CSF but not in blood), and in suspected neoplastic meningitis, when the sugar will be low and malignant cells will be discovered on cytological examination of the sediment. Neurophysiological tests are rarely informative.

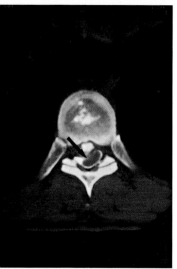

Fig. 164 CT myelogram. Calcified degenerate thoracic disc compressing spinal cord (arrow).

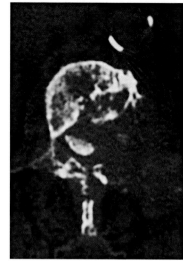

Fig. 165 CT myelogram showing extensive extradural spinal metastatic disease.

Root lesions occur in:

- spondylosis with osteophyte formation encroaching on one or more intervertebral foramina
- prolapse of degenerate disc material, trapping a nerve root in the lateral recess of the spinal canal
- bony metastases or infections
- trauma—fracture or traction injury to nerve roots (usually cervical)
- neurofibromas arising on nerve roots (Figs 163 and 170)
- herpes zoster virus infections (Fig. 166)—the rash follows a dermatomal distribution
- neuralgic amyotrophy—a cervical polyradicular pain syndrome of uncertain aetiology
- cervical ribs—very rare and usually an asymptomatic incidental finding.

Root lesions cause intense shooting pain in the distribution of the affected nerve root (e.g. sciatica), paraesthesias and numbness, often associated with local vertebral symptoms, e.g. neck stiffness or low back pain. Pain is often induced by sneezing, coughing and straining, or during movement and exercise. Look for limitation of movements of the neck or lumbosacral spine, with impaired straight leg raising. Muscle weakness, loss of reflexes and sensory impairment occur in appropriate myotomal and dermatomal distributions. The most common radiculopathies are C5, C6 and C9 in the upper limb and L5 and S1 in the legs. Most are due to intervertebral disc degeneration and herniation; they may be of sudden or gradual onset.

Investigations

Although plain radiographs may detect narrowing of disc spaces, this is not a sensitive investigation. MR or CT imaging of the relevant spinal segments will reveal the anatomy with precision, allowing identification of herniated disc (Fig. 167), canal or foraminal narrowing (Figs 168 and 169) or cancer (Fig. 165). In NF1 multiple neurofibromas may occur (Fig. 170), and these are best revealed by MRI.

Nerve conduction studies are helpful in excluding peripheral neuropathy, and EMG can confirm denervation in a root distribution, thus defining the limits of the lesion.

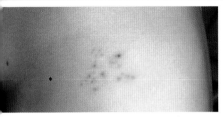

Fig. 166 Shingles (herpes zoster infection); painful, red, vesicular rash in T9 thoracic dermatome.

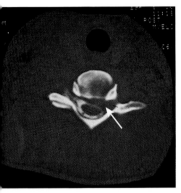

Fig. 167 CT myelogram showing cervical disc prolapse on left, compressing the exiting root and displacing the spinal cord (arrow).

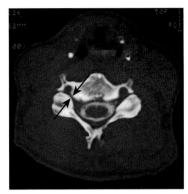

Fig. 168 CT myelogram showing right osteophytic encroachment on nerve root in intervertebral foramen. Compare diameter of neural foramina (arrows) on the two sides.

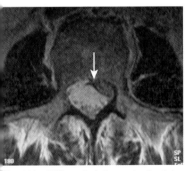

Fig. 169 MRI cervical disc protrusion into spinal canal (arrow).

Management

Most root lesions respond to rest followed by progressive exercise. Analgesic support may be necessary. Traction is a traditional remedy of dubious benefit. Collar immobilization of the neck should be used with caution, except at night, since it can weaken the neck musculature. Rest in bed with a firm mattress provides relief in the initial stages. Once the symptoms have abated, carefully graded exercises with progressive mobilization should ensure continuing clinical improvement. Swimming is an excellent way of building up paravertebral muscle strength. Surgery should be considered if the symptoms, particularly pain, do not respond to medical treatment or if there is progressive muscle weakness, or sensory loss.

Lumbar canal stenosis

A congenitally narrow spinal canal combined with degenerative spondylosis (Fig. 171) and vascular disease presents with lower limb cramps and aches on standing and walking (i.e. with exercise), often with numbness and weakness of the legs. There is usually a long history of low back pain; sphincter disturbance is uncommon. Typically, symptoms remit with rest and spinal flexion, or by flexing the legs at hips and knees. Decompression of the lumbar canal at multiple levels is usually required.

In *cauda equina syndrome* there is spinal stenosis (often spondylotic) with an acute central lumbosacral disc herniation causing severe bilateral sciatic pain, saddle anaesthesia and loss of bladder and bowel control, with very little weakness of ankle musculature but weakness of hip stabilization and hip extension. The ankle jerks may be present. *Turn the patient over and examine buttock sensation and anal sphincter tone.*

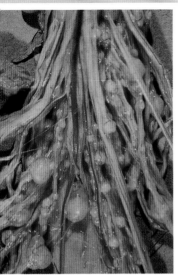

Fig. 170 Postmortem specimen showing multiple neurofibromas of the cauda equina.

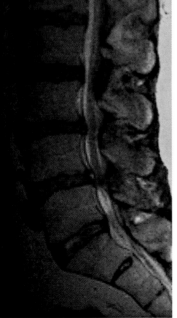

Fig. 171 MRI lumbosacral spine showing hour-glass deformation of spinal canal due to canal stenosis.

32 Developmental abnormalities

Developmental abnormalities

Hydrocephalus

This is the most common easily recognized developmental abnormality. It occurs as a primary abnormality or as a feature of neural tube defects, e.g. in dysraphisms such as spina bifida or with Arnold–Chiari malformation.

In infancy, hydrocephalus (Fig. 172) is usually due to *obstruction* of flow of CSF, often in the aqueduct of Sylvius. *Aqueductal stenosis* causes CSF to accumulate in the lateral and third ventricles, causing dilatation of these ventricles (Fig. 173) and, if decompensated, raised intracranial pressure. *Communicating* hydrocephalus is due to failure of CSF resorption, often following meningitis, head trauma or subarachnoid bleeding, and is therefore commoner in adults. In most patients, however, no cause is evident.

Hydrocephalus develops slowly, presenting in infancy with increasing head size and ocular signs, especially downward deviation at rest (sunset sign) with slight dilation of the pupils. Physical and mental milestones may be delayed, and tone is floppy. Papilloedema is uncommon. Hydrocephalus in adults presents with raised intracranial pressure headache, vomiting and *ataxia*, sometimes with a *frontal dementia* and *incontinence*. The adult head cannot enlarge.

Other developmental abnormalities

Other developmental abnormalities involve the brain itself (e.g. agenesis of the corpus callosum, porencephaly, Fig. 174), probably due to infarction in utero in a vascular territory, and developmental failure of neuronal migration, resulting in cortical dysplasias that may present with epilepsy. Craniofacial malformations, e.g. cleft palate, are usually not accompanied by brain malformations.

Cerebral palsy

Maldevelopment of part of the brain, infarction, perinatal hypoxia or kernicterus causes *cerebral palsy*, a congenital spastic hemiplegia (or diplegia)—often with normal intelligence—which is associated with smallness of the weak limbs (Fig. 175) and seizures. The hemisphere opposite the abnormal limbs is atrophic.

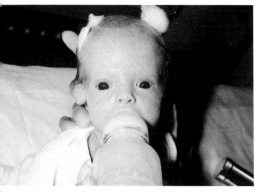

Fig. 172   Infantile hydrocephalus with lid retraction and 'sunset' eye position.

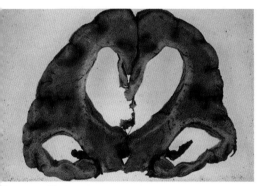

Fig. 173   Dilation of lateral and third ventricles in hydrocephalus due to aqueductal stenosis.

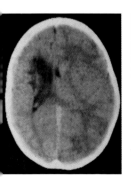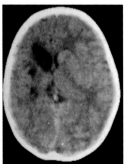

Fig. 174   CT hemiatrophy of the right hemisphere, with a porencephalic cystic cavity in the frontal white matter.

Chiari malformation

In the Chiari malformation, there is elongation of the cerebellar vermis and of the cerebellar tonsils, with herniation of the tonsils and medulla downward into the foramen magnum (Fig. 176). The posterior fossa may be smaller than normal. Hydrocephalus, syringomyelia (Fig. 162) and spina bifida are often associated.

Neurofibromatosis

NF1 is an inherited neurocutaneous syndrome in which *café au lait* spots, freckling and cutaneous nodules consisting of hard and soft (plexiform) neuromas may occur (Fig. 177). The peripheral nerves may be nodular with neurofibromas. Spinal neurofibromas arise on dorsal nerve roots. CNS tumours develop (meningiomas, neurofibromas and gliomas) and tumours of neuroendocrine tissues such as phaeochromocytoma (causing hypertension) occur. Schwannomas particularly occur on cranial nerve VIII, causing unilateral deafness, tinnitus and dizziness. Mental retardation and macrocephaly may be features. The NF1 gene can be tested for diagnosis and genetic counselling.

NF2 has a different genetic basis and tends to cause bilateral VIIIth nerve tumours.

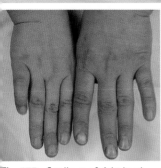

Fig. 175 Smallness of right hand (and arm) due to neonatal hemiplegia.

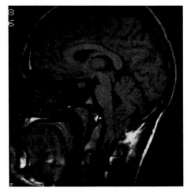

Fig. 176 MRI Chiari malformation. The lower brainstem is elongated, and the tonsils lie in the upper spinal canal below the plane of the foramen magnum.

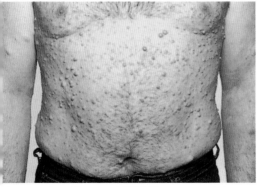

Fig. 177 Neurofibromatosis (NF1). The cutaneous lesions are characteristic.

Head injuries are the commonest cause of disability among young people in contemporary Western societies, occurring as a result of traffic accidents, industrial accidents, domestic accidents, violence, and war injuries. In *closed* head injuries, there is no penetration of the brain's coverings. In *open* head injury, the brain is exposed or penetrated, allowing the possibility of direct injury and infection. Most head injuries are closed. These result in *concussion* or *contusion*, or even in *haemorrhage* into the brain or into the subdural or extradural spaces. *Always exclude an associated injury of the cervical spine* in a head-injured patient.

Concussion

Simple concussion is due to sudden accelerative forces applied to the brain, causing transient distortion of the brain within the cranial cavity. There may be axonal injury (Fig. 178).

Clinical features

The clinical features depend on the forces involved; the severity of the head injury (HI) can be predicted from the occurrence of loss of consciousness (concussion) and the duration of any subsequent post-traumatic amnesia (PTA). PTA less than 30 min is defined as a mild HI, 30 min to 24 hours as moderate HI, and longer than 24 hours as severe HI. In general, head injuries without loss of consciousness do not cause permanent neuropsychiatric sequelae.

Contusion

Cerebral contusion (Fig. 179) occurs from haemorrhage into the brain, usually *contre coup* (opposite) to the site of the injury and most often in the frontal, temporal or occipital regions at the white matter/grey matter junction (Fig. 180).

Clinical features

Contusions are nearly always associated with severe concussive brain injury and carry a high risk of residual cerebral deficit and post-traumatic epilepsy. In fatal closed head injuries, there is a combination of cerebral white matter oedema (due to widespread severe axonal disruption) and contusion.

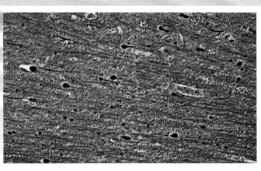

Fig. 178 Closed head injury with axonal injury. The densely argyrophilic blobs represent extruded axoplasmic material from severed axons and associated glial reaction.

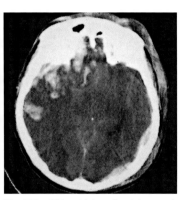

Fig. 179 CT head injury. Frontotemporal contusions shown by focal zones of increased density in subcortical regions of the right side of the brain.

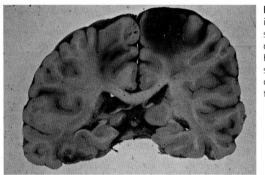

Fig. 180 Fatal head injury. The brain is swollen, with obliteration of the sulci of both hemispheres. There are subcortical haemorrhagic contusions, especially in the left parafalcine region.

Traumatic intracranial haemorrhage

Subdural haematoma (Fig. 181) is due to haemorrhage in the subdural space, usually from a ruptured vein. The haematoma consists of a collection of old and new haemorrhage of variable density (Fig. 181). This expanding mass causes marked lateral and downward shift of the brain, with compression of the lateral ventricles (Fig. 181) and transtentorial herniation (Fig. 182).

Clinical features

Most subdural haematomas are subacute or chronic; there is a delay of hours, days or even weeks before presentation. Headache, confusion and gradual impairment of consciousness, with focal features, e.g. hemiparesis, develop. If the subdural mass continues to expand, transtentorial herniation of the medial temporal lobe will cause compression of the ipsilateral third nerve and impairment of brainstem function. An ipsilateral third nerve palsy develops, with dilation of the pupil followed by ptosis and extraocular muscle weakness. Compression of the contralateral pyramid against the tentorial edge causes hemiplegia on the side of the third nerve palsy (Fig. 182). Later, unless the haematoma is removed, the pontomesencephalic respiratory centres are depressed and death results. If the posterior cerebral artery is compressed against the tentorial edge occipital infarction will occur, causing hemianopia. Haemorrhage in the midbrain (Duret haemorrhages) due to brainstem compression may cause failure to regain consciousness (Fig. 183).

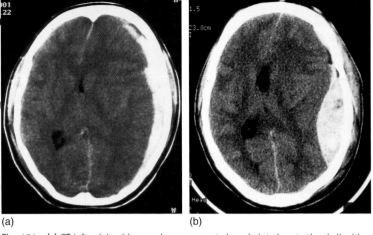

(a)   (b)

Fig. 181 (a) CT left subdural haemorrhage, crescent-shaped clot close to the skull with marked swelling and shift of the brain to the opposite side with compression of the lateral ventricle. (b) CT left extradural haematoma, lens-shaped clot with marked shift of the brain. This may be an acutely developing lesion.

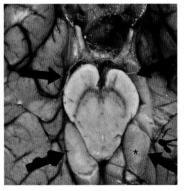

Fig. 182 Uncal herniation through the tentorium. The uncus of both temporal lobes (*) has been squeezed downward through the tentorial notch (arrows), causing compression of the brainstem.

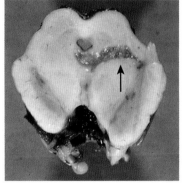

Fig. 183 Midbrain haemorrhages in fatal brainstem compression associated with head injury (arrow).

Clinical features	A *skull fracture* (Fig. 184) increases the chance of the development of intracranial bleeding. If there is a displacement of the fracture into the brain (depressed fracture), this may need surgical debridement. Cortical injury increases the probability of the later development of epilepsy.
	Acute subdural haematoma causes deterioration as described above, but in a few hours; it is due to more rapid and massive haemorrhage, usually with extensive skull fracture.
	Acute extradural haemorrhage is due to bleeding from the middle meningeal artery associated with skull fracture (Fig. 184). Loss of consciousness develops rapidly within a few hours of the accident, or the haematoma is discovered by routine triage scanning in the emergency setting. The patient may recover consciousness after the initial head injury, but then lapse into coma as the haematoma rapidly expands: 'head injuries that talk and die'. Very urgent investigation (CT scan) and aspiration of the haematoma is required.
Management	Urgent surgical assessment is required. Subdural and extradural haematomas should be evacuated at once. Brain contusions are usually managed conservatively. Intracranial pressure monitoring is useful in deciding whether to decompress the swollen brain in closed head injury (Fig. 185). Adequate ventilation, calorie intake and intensive care are essential in the immediate aftermath of the injury. The role of therapeutic hypothermia is still debated.

Spinal cord injuries

The spine may also be injured alone or in association with head injury. Most cervical injuries occur at C5/6 and may cause paraplegia or quadriplegia. It is essential to consider the possibility of an unstable cervical spine fracture in patients complaining of severe pain and stiffness of the neck after head injury. Atlanto-occipital subluxation, where the head is partially dislocated from the top of the spinal column, is rare except in rheumatoid arthritis and ankylosing spondylitis.

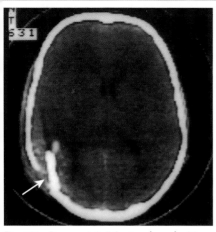

Fig. 184 Depressed skull fracture (arrow) with associated contusional injury.

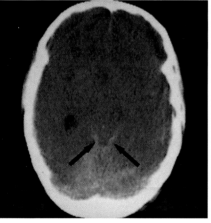

Fig. 185 CT brain scan showing generalized brain swelling with effacement of basal cisterns in a closed head injury (arrows).

Coma is due to brainstem dysfunction; it has many structural and metabolic causes. These include:

- mass lesions, e.g. intracranial haemorrhage, brain infarct, tumour, abscess
- closed head injury
- infections, e.g. meningitis and encephalitis
- epilepsy, e.g. ictal and postictal states
- drug toxicity
- hypo- and hyperglycaemia
- hypoxic encephalopathy
- endocrine disease, including hypopituitarism, hypothyroidism, Addison's disease, hypercalcaemia
- hepatic or renal failure.

Clinical features

Coma is defined according to a simple examination schema that assesses the best verbal response, the best motor response and eye movements—the Glasgow Coma Scale (Fig. 186). The best possible score is 15 and the worst possible score is 3 (not zero). In any patient with altered consciousness it is important to assess the airway, breathing, circulation, level of consciousness and brainstem function (pupils, eye movements, vestibulo-ocular reflexes, the corneal, gag, coughing and swallowing reflexes, rate and rhythm of respiration). Check the neck for rigidity and the limbs for postural tone, spontaneous movements, response to pain and reflexes. Specific causes can often be identified by clinical assessment.

Eye opening		Best verbal response		Best motor response	
Spontaneous	4	Oriented	5	Obeys commands	6
To speech	3	Confused	4	Localizes pain	5
To pain	2	Inappropriate	3	Normal withdrawal	4
None	1	Incomprehensible	2	Abnormal flexion	3
		None	1	Abnormal extension	2
				None	1

Fig. 186 Glasgow Coma Scale (GCS). Note that the minimum score is 3 and the maximum 15. This scale can be used by paramedical and medical staff alike. It is reliable. Clearly, focal lesions causing hemiplegia or aphasia must be recognized separately.

(a) Mid-position fixed pupils in brainstem death

(b) Pinpoint pupils in pontine haemorrhage

(c) Right IIIrd nerve palsy. Dilated unreactive pupil with ptosis. The eye is deviated laterally due to unopposed action of the lateral rectus muscle

Fig. 187 Some pupil signs.

Investigations

These include tests for urea and electrolytes, blood sugar, calcium, liver and renal function and blood gases. Consider drug screen, thyroid tests and cortisol level, MRI or CT (Fig. 185), EEG (Figs 188 and 189) and CSF examination, to exclude infection.

Management

Ensure that the patient is well oxygenated, give intravenous glucose and thiamine, control blood pressure and seizures, treat infections, correct acid–base disturbances and consider naloxone therapy. In intracranial hypertension, give mannitol and hyperventilate. Insertion of an intracranial pressure-measuring bolt is important in ongoing assessment since it may determine the need for medical or surgical treatment.

Management

Brainstem death

Certain clinical criteria based on determination of the absence of brainstem reflexes (respiratory pattern, brain-modified pulse rate variability, loss of temperature control, pupils, caloric responses), absence of motor behaviours other than spinal or brainstem reflex functions, and non-responsive coma are used to determine that irreversible brain death has occurred. Assessment by two experienced physicians, repeated after 12–24 hours, is required. These criteria have been carefully defined by a joint committee of the Royal Colleges and should be very carefully followed. They are generally followed in Europe, North America, Australasia and other Western countries, and have been much used in the process of organ transplantation.

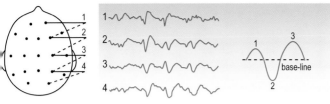

Fig. 188 Triphasic waves seen on EEG in coma resulting from liver failure.

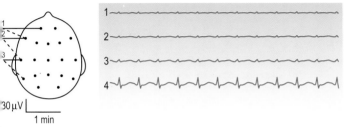

30 μV

1 min

Fig. 189 'Flat EEG'. Isoelectric trace indicating absent brain activity. Channel 4 records the EEG. EEG recordings are not necessary in the diagnosis of brainstem death.

• Two *senior doctors*, one of Consultant grade, must test the patient together

• Wait 6 hours from onset of coma (24 hours if cardiac arrest)
• Exclude CNS depressant drugs, neuromuscular blocking drugs and metabolic or endocrine causes

Tests for absent brainstem function
• Pupil responses absent
• Corneal responses absent
• Eye movements absent to cold caloric testing on each side
• Cranial movements absent to stimulation of face, trunk and limbs
• Gag response absent
• Cough reflex absent

• Recommended tests for apnoea must be carried out
• All respiratory movements must be absent

Fig. 190 Diagnosis of brain death (dependent principally on brainstem tests).

Dementia is a neuropsychiatric disorder resulting in progressive impairment of cognitive function. Although there is usually global cerebral dysfunction, relatively selective syndromes occur, e.g. fronto-temporal dementia and primary progressive aphasic dementia.

Clinical features

The deficits noted vary depending on the underlying aetiology; they include impairment of memory (especially short-term memory and visuo-spatial memory), speech, calculations and other abstractions, writing, orientation and praxis. In *Alzheimer's dementia* there is early loss of spatial memory and autobiographical memory with visual agnosia and loss of numeracy. In *fronto-temporal dementia* personality deterioration is an early feature, with repetitive routines of behaviour and language impairment. In *subcortical dementias*, bradyphrenia and extrapyramidal or corticospinal signs dominate the clinical picture. *Multi-infarct dementia* typically shows a stepwise progression. The MiniMental Status Examination is a useful screening test (Fig. 191).

Aetiology

Always particularly remember treatable conditions (some 15% of the total) and rule out psychiatric disorders (e.g. depression) that may mimic dementia.
  The causes of dementia are:

* *Degenerative:* the most common cause of dementia in patients older than 60 is *Alzheimer's* disease. This degenerative brain disease shows cortical atrophy on MRI (Fig. 192), with senile plaques and neurofibrillary tangles (Fig. 193). Other degenerative dementias include Pick's disease, Huntington's disease, multisystem atrophy and Parkinson's disease.

Orientation	
• What is the time, date (day, month, year)?	5
• What is the name of this ward, hospital, district, town, country?	5
Registration	
• Remember three objects	3
Attention and calculation	
• Subtract 7 from 100 (sequence of five)	5
Recall	
• Ask for recall of the three objects noted above	3
Language	
• Name two objects	2
• Repeat 'no ifs, ands or buts'	1
• Test a three-stage motor command	3
• Test a written motor command	1
• Ask a patient to write a sentence (must contain subject, verb, object)	1
• Test copying of two irregular interlocking pentagons	1

Fig. 191 MiniMental Status Examination (MMSE). Total 30; scores <21 are associated with cognitive impairment (of any cause).

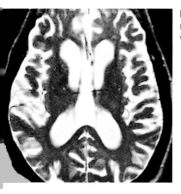

Fig. 192 Alzheimer's dementia with marked cerebral atrophy. Note the dilated ventricles and cerebral sulci.

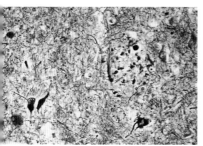

Fig. 193 Alzheimer's disease. Neurofibrillary tangles (right centre) and senile plaques (lower left) in the brain.

Aetiology

- *Vascular:* multiple cerebral infarcts and diffuse small vessel disease. Alzheimer's dementia and vascular disease often coexist (Fig. 194).
- *Neoplastic:* frontal tumours and large meningiomas.
- *Trauma:* chronic subdural haematoma.
- *Infection:* syphilis, Creutzfeldt–Jakob disease, AIDS-related dementia (Fig. 195).
- *Toxic:* alcohol, lead and carbon monoxide, drug intoxication.
- *Metabolic:* hypothyroidism, hepatic failure, uraemia, B_{12} deficiency, prolonged hypoglycaemia and prolonged hypoxia.
- *Paraneoplastic encephalopathies:* especially limbic encephalitis presenting with an amnesic syndrome.
- *Psychiatric:* depression may cause a treatable pseudo-dementia.

Management

Once treatable causes have been eliminated, management is largely supportive. Patients with dementia cause considerable strain on their immediate family and eventually institutional care may be required.

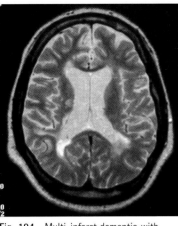

Fig. 194 Multi-infarct dementia with cerebral atrophy.

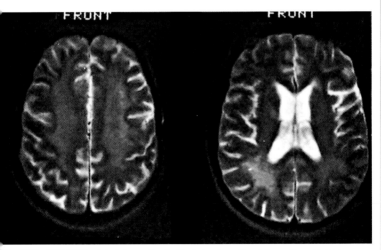

Fig. 195 MRI AIDS-related dementia. Cortical atrophy with white matter changes suggestive of progressive multifocal leukoencephalopathy (PML). Diffuse and focal white matter change in T2 weighted scan.

Headache and facial pain are probably the commonest clinical problems in neurological practice. These symptoms may be due to serious disease, e.g. raised intracranial pressure, meningitis or giant cell arteritis (Fig. 196), or to abnormalities within the orbits, ears or sinuses, especially infection (Fig. 197) and neoplasms, and dental disease. Most headaches are benign and fall into one of three categories: tension-type headache, migraine and cluster headaches. The most common headache is tension-type headache. Women are generally more prone to headache than men.

Clinical types

Tension-type headache
Generalized headache, often starting occipitally and radiating over the vertex and around the head either in a tight band or as a heavy pressure. It can be nearly continuous for long periods of time, even years, or intermittent. It varies from week to week and day to day, and is often clearly related to personal or environmental stress. Examination may reveal localized tenderness in pericranial muscles and skin.

Management Reassurance, often requiring neuroimaging, is usually helpful. Time spent in exploring possible stressors is time well spent. The importance of sparing use of analgesics should be explained, and a nocturnal tricyclic antidepressant may effectively interrupt the headache sequence.

Migraine
Characterized by attacks of headache lasting a few hours or days. A chronic, near-continuous form occurs. Onset is usually in adolescence. Typically, there is a recurrent, unilateral, throbbing frontotemporal ache associated with nausea, photophobia, phonophobia and irritability. It is worsened by physical activity. It is more common in women and often there is a family history. In classic attacks, the pain is preceded by visual phenomena. Temporary focal neurological signs including hemianopia, hemiplegia or hemisensory loss may occur. Focal features should suggest the need for neuroimaging. Retinal migraine with unilateral visual symptoms occurs. Cerebral infarction may rarely complicate a migraine attack. Other variants include migraine without aura.

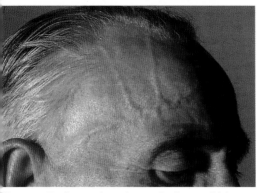

Fig. 196 Swollen, tender and non-pulsatile superficial temporal artery in giant cell arteritis.

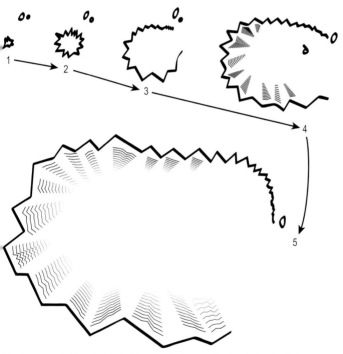

Fig. 197 Evolution of fortification spectra in the visual field in classical migraine. The visual 'teichopsia' develop over a few minutes in central vision of both eyes and extend in size before gradually resolving. There is a flickering quality to the visual disturbance and a striking linearity to its edges. It is the result of brief cortical dysfunction caused by spreading depression across the visual cortex (1–5).

Management Tricyclic antidepressants or beta-blockers may be helpful in prophylaxis. Triptans are effective in relieving an acute attack. Ergotamine is now little used. Simple analgesics should be used sparingly.

Cluster headache
Characterized by clusters of episodic, severe pain in and around one eye and cheek. Typically, attacks last 20 min to 2 h, occur once or twice daily (often at night) over a period of weeks and are associated with reddening/watering of the eye, stuffiness of the nose and nasal mucous discharge. The syndrome is more common in men and sometimes precipitated by alcohol.

Management Acute episodes respond to sumatriptan. Valproate is sometimes useful as a prophylactic, and methysergide is effective, at the risk, like many ergot derivatives, of inducing retroperitoneal and pericardial fibrosis. High-flow oxygen inhalation is also helpful in refractory cases.

SUNCT
Short-lasting unilateral neuralgiform pain with conjunctival congestion and tearing; attacks of pain and redness of the eye without other symptoms lasting only 5–240 s. Often associated with migraine. It may be related to 'ice-pick pain'—brief stabs of pain in the first division of the trigeminal innervation.

Management Indometacin, valproate and lamotrigine may be helpful.

Orgasmic pain (coital cephalalgia)
A syndrome of sudden-onset pain resembling the pain of subarachnoid haemorrhage occurring during sexual intercourse. It is rarely repeated more than once, and its aetiology is unknown. Neuroimaging is indicated to exclude serious cause. *Thunderclap headache* is a similar disorder that occurs without situational factors, that also requires imaging to exclude intracranial pathology.

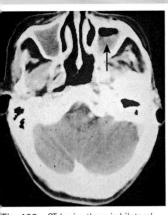

Fig. 198 CT brain; there is bilateral antral opacification due to sinusitis, with an air–fluid level on the left. The patient presented with headache.

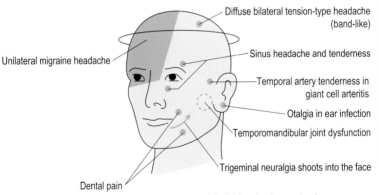

Fig. 199 Location of various common cranial and facial head aches and pains.

Diffuse bilateral tension-type headache (band-like)

Sinus headache and tenderness

Unilateral migraine headache

Temporal artery tenderness in giant cell arteritis

Otalgia in ear infection

Temporomandibular joint dysfunction

Trigeminal neuralgia shoots into the face

Dental pain

Clinical types

Facial pain

Trigeminal neuralgia is a short-lasting (seconds), unilateral, lancinating or shooting pain, usually experienced in the third division of the trigeminal nerve. It is often induced by contact with the cheek or mouth. It affects people in middle life or older, and is often caused by pressure on the proximal part of the trigeminal sensory root by an adjacent cerebellar artery—a branch of the basilar artery (Fig. 200). Less commonly, trigeminal pain may occur in multiple sclerosis and with neurofibroma on the sensory root.

Management   Treatment with carbamazepine or gabapentin is often successful, but benefit may not be maintained. Surgical exploration of the nerve to free it from its proximity to arterial pulsation is usually curative.

Dental pain

Pain in the face or jaw may occur from dental abscess or caries. The affected teeth are usually tender to light tapping or pressure, or during mastication.

Atypical facial pain

Diffuse chronic aching pain in the face may occur with depression. It responds to antidepressant drug therapy.

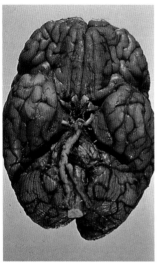

Fig. 200 Ectatic basilar artery causing pressure on the trigeminal nerve root, sometimes the cause of trigeminal neuralgia.

Disorders of stance and gait are a common cause of disability and of injury from accidents and falls. Gait depends on the skeleton and joints to provide stability and fulcrum, muscles to provide power and the nervous system to provide control, including sensory input, a central processing and integrating system, and an efferent system to instruct the muscles.

Aetiology and classification

Disorders of gait may have orthopaedic, muscular or neurological causes, or be due to local pain.
   Neurological causes include:

- large fibre sensory neuropathy, with loss of joint position sense
- dorsal column degeneration (e.g. vitamin B_{12} deficiency), multiple sclerosis, paraneoplastic degeneration, hepatic disease and tabes dorsalis
- inner ear disease, e.g. epidemic labyrinthitis (benign positional vertigo)
- brainstem disease involving the vestibular nucleus and its connections
- spastic gait disorders
- cerebellar gait disorders
- frontal gait disorders (apraxic gait)
- Parkinson's disease and other extrapyramidal gait disorders
- drug effects
- falls in the elderly; these are of multiple causation.

Spastic gait disorder: characterized by a narrow-based, short-stepped, lurching gait, with poor elevation of toe and forefoot, so that the toes seem to catch on the ground (Fig. 201). Balance is relatively good and a short-stepped hobbling run may be possible. Spastic circumduction, and a scissoring gait with bilateral spasticity, is characteristic.

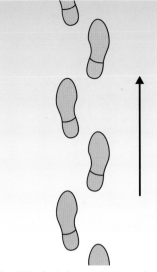

Fig. 201 Foot placement pattern of spastic gait disorder. Note the narrow base and the short steps.

Aetiology and classification

Cerebellar gait disorder: causes a wide-based gait of irregular cadence with a tendency to fall, especially when turning. There is a wandering quality to the gait, in any direction, caused by irregularity in length, direction and rhythm of the steps. The gait of acute alcohol intoxication is a well-known example (Fig. 202).

Parkinsonian gait disorder: has an accelerating quality, with small steps, a rigidity of posture in a flexed stance and an inability to change rhythm or frequency of the gait pattern (Fig. 203). 'Festinant gait'.

Frontal gait disorder: the feet are 'magnetically' attracted to the ground. The gait shows short, rapid, shuffling steps and freezing in mid-task. There is often marked hesitation and disequilibrium. This gait disorder is sometimes described as 'apraxic' since it appears the patient has lost central control mechanisms for 'running the motor program for walking'.

Myopathic gait disorder: shows bilateral hip weakness with Trendelenburg floppiness of hip posture and an exaggerated lumbar lordosis.

Peripheral neuropathy: causes a high steppage gait because there is distal weakness causing foot drop.

Tabes dorsalis and other posterior column sensory disorders: cause a stamping high steppage gait, due to the requirement to increase sensory input by striking the feet hard on the ground.

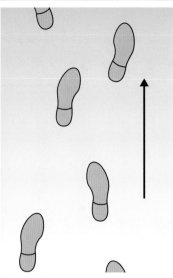

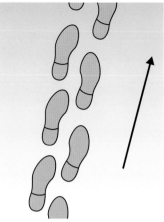

Fig. 203 Foot placement pattern of Parkinson's disease. Note the short overlapping gait cadence.

Fig. 202 Foot placement pattern of cerebellar gait disorder. The foot placement pattern is wide-based and irregular, resembling the pattern of cerebellar disease. In sensory neuropathy, the disorder is markedly worsened by eye closure, which removes visual cues on which the patient is reliant.

? Questions

1. A 58-year-old insulin-dependent diabetic man woke with a severe weakness and impairment of sensation affecting his left arm. Which of the following are appropriate?

a. An emergency cerebral CT scan.
b. Nerve conduction studies to exclude a carpal tunnel syndrome.
c. A blood sugar to exclude hypoglycaemia.
d. Thrombolysis if a cerebral haemorrhage is excluded.
e. Treatment with soluble aspirin.

2. Which of the following are associated with myotonic dystrophy?

a. Sensitivity to the cold.
b. Diabetes mellitus.
c. Insomnia.
d. Cardiomyopathy.
e. Hirsutism.

3. A 70-year-old man presents with a progressive gait disturbance. Neurological examination demonstrates spasticity in both legs. Which of the following are appropriate?

a. MRI of brain to exclude a parasagittal meningioma.
b. MRI of cervical spine to exclude a spinal cord compression.
c. MRI of the lumbar spine to exclude a spinal cord compression.
d. MRI of the thoracic spine to exclude a spinal cord compression.
e. Nerve conduction studies to investigate a possible Guillain–Barré syndrome.

4. A 30-year-old German tourist presents with a right-sided lower motor neuron facial weakness. Which of the following are correct?

a. The absence of a rash excludes Lyme disease.
b. Impairment of taste suggests involvement of the nerve to stapedius.
c. An additional right-sided abducens palsy suggests a cerebello-pontine angle lesion.
d. A course of steroids is indicated in Bell's palsy.
e. Crocodile tears may be a long-term complication of Bell's palsy.

5. In optic disc swelling which of the following are correct?

a. Impaired visual acuity suggests optic neuritis rather than papilloedema.
b. Enlargement of the blind spot is characteristic of papilloedema.
c. In papilloedema transient blindness following exercise warrants urgent treatment.
d. A lumbar puncture should not be performed unless a CT scan has been shown to be normal.
e. In pseudotumour cerebri lumbar puncture is contraindicated.

6. A 60-year-old man dependent on alcohol presents with progressive visual failure. Visual fields suggest a bitemporal hemianopia. Which of the following is correct?

a. A CT or MRI scan is essential in the investigation of a pituitary tumour.
b. An elevated serum prolactin suggests a pituitary tumour.
c. A raised serum cyanide is characteristic of tobacco amblyopia.
d. Visual failure is unlikely to improve following the removal of a pituitary tumour.
e. A suprasellar meningioma can also cause a bitemporal visual field defect.

7. A 36-year-old man presents with a sudden severe headache and double vision. He had meningism and a right-sided third nerve palsy. Which of the following is correct?

a. A normally reacting pupil excludes a posterior communicating artery aneurysm.
b. A CT angiogram is likely to demonstrate a posterior communicating artery aneurysm.
c. The clinical presentation suggests temporal arteritis.
d. Diabetes mellitus is a recognized cause of a painful third nerve palsy.
e. The headache and ptosis is in keeping with migrainous neuralgia.

8. Which of the following usually suggest a left hemisphere tumour?

a. A progressive fluent dysphasia.
b. Dressing apraxia.
c. Adversive seizures with head turning to the left.
d. Progressive spastic dysarthria.
e. Progressive wasting and weakness of the right calf.

9. Wasting of the intrinsic hand muscles commonly occurs in which of the following?

a. Diabetes.
b. Hereditary sensory motor neuropathy
c. Cervical spondylosis.
d. Dermatomyositis.
e. Cerebral palsy.

10. A 56-year-old woman failed to breathe spontaneously following an anaesthetic for a cholecystectomy. Which of the following is applicable?

a. An edrophonium (Tensilon) test is positive in myasthenia gravis.
b. High-dose steroid therapy is indicated in myasthenic patients not responding to anticholinesterases.
c. An edrophonium (Tensilon) test is a simple and safe method of monitoring the dosage of anticholinesterase treatment in myasthenia gravis.
d. In myasthenia gravis increased neuromuscular jitter is a characteristic neurophysiological finding on muscle sampling.
e. IVIg is the treatment of choice in severe myasthenia gravis.

11. Treatment with L-dopa and a dopa decarboxylase inhibitor has been started on a 73-year-old man with suspected Parkinson's disease. He has not improved. Which of the following is appropriate?

a. Failure to improve suggests the diagnosis is incorrect.
b. Postural hypotension is a complication of treatment with L-dopa.
c. Visual hallucinations are suggestive of Lewy body disease.
d. Of the main features of Parkinson's disease, tremor is the least responsive to L-dopa.
e. Akinesia is the most disabling feature of Parkinson's disease.

12. A 70-year-old man presents with a 6-month history of progressive memory loss. Which is correct?

a. B_{12} deficiency is an important treatable cause.
b. A Herxheimer reaction is a dangerous complication of treating neurosyphilis with penicillin.
c. If hypothyroidism is confirmed he should be vigorously treated with high-dose thyroxine.
d. Examination of the spinal fluid may show specific abnormalities diagnostic of Alzheimer's disease.
e. Treatment with cholinergic drugs may be useful in the treatment of both Alzheimer's disease and multi-infarct dementia.

13. A 40-year-old man presents with double vision. Which of the following is appropriate?

a. Double vision persisting with one eye closed suggests a functional cause.
b. Horizontal separation of the images on lateral gaze is likely to be due to a sixth nerve palsy.
c. Myasthenia is an important underlying cause.
d. The outermost image is always the false image.
e. A sixth nerve palsy may not be a reliable localizing sign.

14. A 51-year-old man presents with a lower motor neuron facial weakness. Which of the following is correct?

a. In Bell's palsy hyperacusis is due to involvement of the nerve to stapedius.
b. With an additional sixth nerve palsy the lesion is within the brainstem.
c. An absent corneal reflex suggests a lesion in the cerebello-pontine angle.
d. Crocodile tears are a long-term complication of Bell's palsy.
e. Lyme disease should be considered in patients from Hampshire.

15. A 78-year-old hypertensive lady experienced three episodes of sudden transient loss of vision in the left eye. She has bilateral carotid bruits and is in atrial fibrillation. Which of the following is correct?

a. Aspirin is the treatment of choice.
b. Transient unilateral blindness suggests vascular disease in vertebro-basilar territory.
c. Cholesterol emboli may be seen on fundoscopic examination.
d. She has a risk of permanent dysphasia and hemiplegia.
e. A 50% stenosis at the origin of the internal carotid artery is an indication for endarterectomy or stenting.

16. A 43-year-old lorry driver presents with generalized tonic–clonic seizures heralded by olfactory hallucinations. Which is appropriate?

a. If he refuses to notify the vehicle licensing authority his doctor may do so.
b. An MRI scan is unlikely to demonstrate an intracranial structural lesion.
c. An EEG is an investigation of choice.
d. If a sphenoidal ridge meningioma is removed his epilepsy will be cured and he will no longer require anticonvulsant therapy.
e. Phenytoin is the anticonvulsant of choice.

17. An 80-year-old man presents with progressive unsteadiness of gait. He has become incontinent of urine and his memory is deteriorating. Which of the following is correct?

a. Dilatation of the lateral ventricles without cortical atrophy on the CT scan suggests a hydrocephalus.
b. His gait may improve temporarily with the removal of 30 ml of CSF.
c. A gait disturbance in addition to dementia is typical of Alzheimer's disease.
d. He may improve following the insertion of a ventriculo-peritoneal shunt.
e. Communicating hydrocephalus may be a complication of a previous head injury.

18. In petit mal epilepsy, which of the following are correct?

a. An affected child's school performance may be impaired.
b. Phenytoin is the drug of choice.
c. Attacks may be induced by hyperventilation.
d. Attacks are likely to continue throughout life.
e. 3 per second spike and wave discharges on the EEG are diagnostic.

19. A 68-year-old lady presents with a 3-week history of headache. Which of the following features suggest raised intracranial pressure?

a. Worsening of headache by straining.
b. Episodic headache preceded by visual teichopsia.
c. Scalp tenderness.
d. Neck stiffness.
e. Indistinct disc margins on fundoscopy.

20. A 40-year-old man presents with back pain radiating down his right leg. There is weakness of dorsiflexion of the right foot. Which of the following is correct?

a. In sciatica pain is experienced in a dermatome.
b. The ankle jerk is expected to be absent on the right side.
c. The finding of a prolapsed intervertebral disc on an MRI scan of the lumbar spine is an indication for surgery.
d. Bladder dysfunction is an indication for surgery.
e. An S1 disc prolapse is expected on the MRI scan.

21. A 55-year-old lady presents with progressive weakness of the shoulders and hips. Her muscles are painful and her serum CK is 26000 units. Which of the following is relevant?

a. An underlying neoplasm is likely.
b. A muscle biopsy demonstrates muscle atrophy.
c. High-dose steroids is the treatment of choice.
d. Muscle sampling at EMG shows neurogenic changes.
e. The patient has a Trendelenburg gait.

22. While being investigated for a 5-year history of intermittent headaches preceded by visual teichopsia and nausea, a 42-year-old lady developed an abrupt right-sided weakness and dysphasia. Which is likely?

a. A cerebral CT scan and subsequent MRA study demonstrates a large right hemisphere arterio-venous malformation.
b. A cerebral CT scan demonstrates a left hemisphere metastasis.
c. A CT scan demonstrates a cerebral infarct in her left hemisphere.
d. As the CT scan is normal, the frequency of the patient's headaches should be reduced with prophylactic beta-blockers.
e. The fact that the patient has classical migraine is not relevant when investigating the cause of the dominant hemisphere cerebral infarction.

23. A 27-year-old man presents with headaches provoked by coughing. On examination he has jerk nystagmus, the fast component of which is in a downward direction. The reflexes in the upper limbs are absent, but in the lower limbs the tendon reflexes are brisk with bilateral extensor plantar responses. Which is appropriate?

a. He is likely to have the dissociated sensory loss typical of syringomyelia.
b. A hydrocephalus is likely.
c. Unsteadiness of gait and incontinence would suggest a hydrocephalus.
d. A suspended sensory loss involving the upper limbs and chest would suggest an intramedullary lesion of the cervical cord.
e. Absent reflexes in the upper limbs suggest a peripheral neuropathy.

24. A 50-year-old man presented with failing vision. His feet had increased in size, his wedding ring had become tight and he had recently been found to be diabetic. Which of the following are applicable?

a. A bilateral upper altitudinal visual field is common.
b. A bitemporal visual field defect denotes chiasmal compression.
c. Histology from the trans-sphenoid hypophysectomy demonstrated a basophile adenoma.
d. Carpal tunnel syndromes are due to insulin antagonism.
e. A cardiomyopathy may be fatal.

25. A 49-year-old man was taken to the Accident and Emergency Department, unconscious, having fallen from a ladder. When first seen he was confused but awake, but during the examination his left pupil was observed to dilate as he slipped into a coma. Which are applicable?

a. The lucid interval following the head injury suggests an extradural haematoma.
b. A third nerve palsy suggests coning.
c. He is likely to have sustained a serious cervical injury.
d. The dilated pupil suggests a sixth nerve palsy.
e. The middle meningeal artery may have been damaged.

26. A 22-year-old lady has a long history of focal seizures starting with shaking of the left hand spreading proximally to involve the whole arm before loss of consciousness. Which of the following is true?

a. The left hand being smaller than the right suggests a congenital abnormality.
b. It would be unlikely for her seizures to be due to a cerebral tumour.
c. A left-sided meningioma is likely.
d. An MRI scan shows a right hemisphere astrocytoma.
e. Phenytoin is the anticonvulsant of choice.

27. A 70-year-old lady presents with a constant occipital headache and tenderness of the scalp. A CT scan was normal. The ESR was 105 mm in one hour. Which of the following is true?

a. A normal temporal artery biopsy excludes temporal arteritis.
b. Double vision is a common complication of temporal arteritis.
c. Aching of the shoulders and thighs suggests polymyalgia rheumatica.
d. With high-dose steroids clinical improvement is expected within 48 hours.
e. If blindness occurs it is unlikely that it will recover.

28. A 52-year-old lady, a smoker, presents with double vision, shortness of breath on effort and variable weakness of the shoulder girdle. Which is appropriate?

a. Brisk reflexes are characteristic of myasthenia gravis.
b. Double vision is typical of the Lambert–Eaton syndrome.
c. Thyroid dysfunction may disrupt the control of myasthenia.
d. Anti-MUSK antibodies may be important if acetylcholine receptor antibodies are negative.
e. Absent reflexes suggest Lambert–Eaton myasthenic syndrome (LEMS).

29. A 68-year-old man presented with a 6-month history of progressive pain in both legs induced by exercise. After walking more than 50 yards he would have to stop because of pain in both calves and sometimes he also had pain in the right thigh. He had a long history of intermittent back pain and left-sided sciatica. No abnormality was found on examination. Which of the following are appropriate?

a. Abnormal physical signs in the lower limbs may well be found if he is examined after he has walked 50 yards on the flat.
b. Abnormal physical signs in the lower limbs are more likely to be found if examined after climbing three flights of stairs.
c. Despite preserved ankle reflexes, the MRI scan of the lumbar spine shows a prolapsed disc embarrassing the L4 nerve roots.
d. Because of the long history of back pain, surgical decompression is unlikely to be successful.
e. Claudication of the cauda equina may be associated with a spinal AVM.

30. Progressive myoclonus may be associated with:

a. Metabolic disorders including Gaucher's disease.
b. Subacute sclerosing panencephalitis.
c. Diabetes.
d. Motor neuron disease.
e. Creutzfeldt–Jakob disease.

31. For 6 months a 60–year–old lady complained of burning pains in the left thigh. She had injured her back several years previously in a road traffic accident. At times she experienced tingling with some numbness in both feet. On examination the ankle jerks were absent. She was obese and a rash in both groins suggested a fungal infection. Which of the following are appropriate?

a. If she has a prolapsed lumbar disc at L4/L5 her symptoms may be relieved by weight loss.
b. Her symptoms may be due to compression of the lateral cutaneous nerve of the thigh.
c. Meralgia paraesthetica may be the first presentation of diabetes.
d. Nerve conduction studies may show absent sural nerve action potentials as evidence of a peripheral neuropathy.
e. Following a local anaesthetic into the lateral cutaneous nerve of the thigh, the patient could be left with an uncomfortable numbness in the thigh.

32. A 23-year-old housewife developed pain in the left eye and became sensitive to light. The left pupil was large and unreactive to light. Which of the following are likely?

a. In the absence of ptosis a third nerve palsy is still the most likely diagnosis.
b. Sympathetic overactivity reflects a Horner's syndrome.
c. Absent reflexes in the lower limbs are to be expected.
d. The pupil should constrict in response to a sustained light stimulus.
e. Preserved tendon reflexes excludes a myotonic pupil.

33. A 58-year-old man presents with a tremor of the upper limbs. Which of the following are true?

a. A postural tremor may be drug induced.
b. An asymmetric resting tremor is unusual in Parkinson's disease.
c. Beta-blockers may be useful in the treatment of benign essential tremor.
d. Parkinsonian tremor responds well to L-dopa and dopa agonists.
e. His past history of in-patient psychiatric treatment may be important.

34. A 55-year-old lady presents with vertigo and unsteadiness. Which of the following are important?

a. Nausea and vomiting suggests the vertigo is peripheral in origin.
b. Dysarthria and weakness of the limbs suggests vertebrobasilar ischaemia.
c. Vertigo on neck extension is common in cervical spondylosis.
d. Vertigo provoked by putting either ear down to the pillow suggests a peripheral cause.
e. The Epley manoeuvre will suppress central vertigo.

35. A 58-year-old man presents with pain, wasting and weakness of the left thigh. The quadriceps is wasted and weak. The left knee jerk and both ankle jerks are absent. Which of the following are relevant?

a. The absence of back pain excludes a prolapsed lumbar intervertebral disc.
b. A blood sugar estimation may be relevant.
c. The weakness of extension of the knee is likely to be due to a pyramidal (an upper motor neuron) lesion.
d. Diabetic amyotrophy is due to a lesion of the femoral nerve.
e. This distribution of wasting and weakness is typical of an L4/5 prolapsed intervertebral disc.

36. Which of the following are associated with hypothyroidism?

a. Ataxia of gait.
b. Amenorrhoea.
c. Deafness.
d. Dementia.
e. Psychosis.

37. A 40-year-old man has had problems with his walking since his teens. His father and younger brother have similar problems. Like his brother, he too has wasted hands and calves. They, like their father, have pes cavus. Which of the following are true?

a. A slowing of motor conduction velocity denotes a demyelinating peripheral neuropathy.
b. Immunosuppression may slow the progression of disability.
c. Preservation of tendon reflexes suggests an axonal neuropathy.
d. Type 2 hereditary sensory motor neuropathy (HSMN) is characterized by demyelination of the peripheral nerves.
e. Type 1 HSMN is due to an axonal neuropathy.

38. A 60-year-old lady failed to recover consciousness after a general anaesthetic for surgery to her varicose veins. She is on a life support system in the intensive care unit. Which of the following are correct?

a. Irrecoverable brain damage has not occurred if ice-cold water introduced into the external auditory meatus induces nystagmus with a fast phase towards the cold stimulus.
b. The oculo-cephalic reflex may be abolished in patients receiving sedation.
c. Cold water introduced into the external auditory canal induces tonic deviation of the eyes towards the cold stimulus in unconscious patients with preserved brainstem activity.
d. Tests for irreversible brain death are unreliable in patients with hypothermia.
e. An EEG is essential for the diagnosis of irreversible brain death.

39. A 68-year-old lady presents with episodes of severe facial pain affecting the right lower jaw. Which of the following are correct?

a. If a rash complicates treatment with carbamazepine, trials of other anticonvulsants may be of benefit.
b. An absent corneal reflex suggests a lesion of the cerebello-pontine angle.
c. Lancinating pains affecting the upper face are unusual in idiopathic trigeminal neuralgia.
d. Trigeminal neuralgia may occur in younger patients with multiple sclerosis.
e. Trigeminal neuralgia may be a complication of diabetes.

40. In suspected meningitis which of the following are appropriate?

a. In a sterile spinal fluid a very low CSF sugar may be suggestive of malignant meningitis.
b. A low spinal fluid sugar occurs in bacterial meningitis.
c. In meningitis it is unwise to perform a lumbar puncture without ensuring a CT scan is normal.
d. A purpuric rash suggests *Haemophilus influenzae* infection.
e. Cryptococcal meningitis may complicate immune deficiency disorders.

41. In multiple sclerosis which of the following are correct?

a. Beta-interferon slows the clinical progression in patients with primary progressive disease.
b. MS may present with a progressive spastic paraparesis.
c. Beta-interferon reduces the eventual disability in patients with relapsing and remitting disease.
d. Steroids curtail clinical relapses but do not alter ultimate disability.
e. Disability may transiently deteriorate with exercise.

42. A 28-year-old man presents with excessive episodic daytime sleepiness. Which of the following are correct?

a. In narcolepsy nocturnal sleep is usually interrupted.
b. Dream recall is better if patients are woken during deep stage 4 sleep rather than if woken during REM sleep.
c. Transient nocturnal paralysis suggests underlying epilepsy with Todd's paresis.
d. Episodes of collapse in situations evoking strong emotions suggest hysteria.
e. Associated symptoms of the narcolepsy syndrome respond well to dexamfetamine.

43. A 63-year-old lady presents with a progressive ataxia. Which of the following could be relevant?

a. Specific chromosomal studies to confirm the diagnosis of Friedreich's ataxia.
b. Full investigations to exclude an occult malignancy.
c. Cortisol levels to exclude Addison's disease.
d. Thyroid function tests to exclude Graves' disease.
e. MRI scanning to investigate the possibility of multiple sclerosis.

44. Which of the following are recognized as non–metastatic manifestations of malignant disease?

a. Amyotrophic lateral sclerosis.
b. A predominantly sensory neuropathy.
c. Spinal cord compression.
d. Myasthenia gravis.
e. Painful muscular weakness.

45. A CSF protein >1 g per 100 ml with no cellular increase may occur in:

a. A spinal cord compression.
b. Tuberculosis.
c. Meningococcal meningitis.
d. Acoustic neurinoma.
e. Guillain–Barré syndrome.

46. Which of the following may be associated with a bitemporal hemianopsia?

a. Craniopharyngioma.
b. Pituitary adenoma.
c. A glioma involving the left temporal lobe.
d. A posterior communicating artery aneurysm.
e. Tobacco–alcohol amblyopia.

47. A 23-year-old lady was struck in the neck during a robbery. Several days later she developed weakness of the left face, arm and leg. Which of the following are relevant?

a. A right-sided Horner's syndrome suggests occlusion of the internal carotid artery.
b. A long previous history of intermittent headaches suggests cerebral infarction complicating migraine.
c. An MRA study is important to exclude a dissection of the internal carotid artery.
d. A normal CT scan implies no serious intracranial pathology and suggests the patient is seeking compensation.
e. Anticoagulation with warfarin is the treatment of choice in carotid artery dissection.

48. A 30-year-old man presents with a sudden onset headache with neck stiffness. Which of the following is correct?

a. Hydrocephalus is a common complication of subarachnoid haemorrhage.
b. A third nerve palsy suggests anterior communicating artery aneurysm.
c. Confusion and lower limb weakness suggests vascular spasm in anterior cerebral artery territory.
d. Cerebral aneurysms may be familial.
e. Incidental aneurysms of less than 10 mm in diameter pose a particular risk for haemorrhage.

49. A 65-year-old man presents with progressive short-term memory loss. Which of the following is relevant?

a. Nystagmus and absent ankle jerks suggest Korsakoff's psychosis.
b. Small unreacting pupils with a neuropathic ankle joint suggest an infective cause for the dementia.
c. Nowadays HIV testing is relevant.
d. Thyrotoxicosis is a treatable cause of dementia.
e. Anticholinergic drugs may be important in the treatment of Alzheimer's disease.

50. A 72-year-old man presents with a 3-month history of progressive confusion, often becoming lost in familiar surroundings. Which of the following is appropriate?

a. A CT scan is likely to show a right hemisphere cerebral infarction.
b. Dressing apraxia is further evidence of a non-dominant parietal lesion.
c. Coincidental dysphasia would suggest cerebral metastases.
d. Headaches would suggest temporal arteritis.
e. A right hemisphere tumour is likely.

Answers

1. (see sections 14, 15)

Correct answers: a, c, d
The sudden onset of neurological deficit suggests vascular disease, transient ischaemic attack (TIA) or completed stroke, in this case in right middle cerebral artery territory. An emergency CT scan (a) is essential to determine whether the lesion is due to cerebral infarction or haemorrhage, particularly if thrombolytic therapy is being considered. Hypoglycaemia must be excluded in diabetic patients presenting with acute neurological disease (c) since, if unrecognized, it can result in permanent disability. If cerebral haemorrhage has been excluded, thrombolysis is the treatment of choice provided it can be given within 3 hours of the onset of stroke (d).

Incorrect answers: b, e
The history does not suggest carpal tunnel syndrome (b). Aspirin, important in stroke prevention, is possibly helpful, but not essential in acute stroke resuscitation (e).

2. (see section 26)

Correct answers: a, b, d
Patients with myotonic dystrophy typically find their muscle stiffness (due to myotonia) is worse when they are exposed to cold (a). Mild diabetes is often associated with myotonic dystrophy (b), and cardiomyopathy may lead to heart failure (d).

Incorrect answers: c, e
Patients with myotonic dystrophy complain of hypersomnia, not insomnia (c). Hirsutism is not a feature of myotonic dystrophy, but it is associated with gonadal failure (e).

3. (see section 30)

Correct answers: b, d
The clinical picture is that of a spastic paraplegia. Urgent investigation must aim to exclude spinal cord compression, e.g. due to prolapsed intervertebral disc or intraspinal tumour, benign or malignant (b and d). Delayed surgical decompression risks permanent neurological disability and bladder dysfunction.

Incorrect answers: a, c, e
Spastic paraparesis is only very rarely due to parasagittal meningioma (a). Cervical or thoracic spinal cord lesion is likely. Leg weakness due to lumbar disc disease is of LMN type, as the lesion is below (caudal to) the termination of the spinal cord (c). The history is not that of a Guillain–Barré syndrome (e).

4. (see section 8)

Correct answers: d, e
A short course of corticosteroids may hasten the recovery of Bell's palsy (d). Aberrant regeneration of nerve fibres frequently develops because nerve fibres which previously innervated the salivary glands may reroute via the greater superficial petrosal nerve to the otic ganglion to innervate the lacrimal gland, resulting in 'crocodile tears' on the affected side when the patient is exposed to the sight or smell of food (e).

Incorrect answers: a, b, c
Although Lyme disease may cause lower motor neuron facial weakness, the typical rash, erythema migrans, is not invariably present (a). Impairment of taste in the anterior two-thirds of the tongue is due to involvement of the cauda tympani nerve, not the nerve to stapedius (b). A coexisting abducens palsy implies a lesion in the pons, not in the cerebello-pontine angle (c).

5. (see section 1)

Correct answers: a, b, c, d
Early impaired visual acuity is typical of inflammatory disease of the optic nerve (papillitis). In papilloedema, visual acuity is typically preserved (a). Enlargement of the blind spot is characteristic of papilloedema (b). Obscuration of vision induced by exercise may herald permanent visual loss (c). It is important to confirm the CT scan is normal before a lumbar puncture to avoid transtentorial coning, which might occur if there is a mass lesion in a cerebral hemisphere (d).

Incorrect answers: e
Lumbar puncture is important in the diagnosis and treatment of benign intracranial hypertension.

6. (see sections 1 and 20)

Correct answers: a, b, c, e
Scanning, CT and MRI, is essential in the diagnosis of pituitary tumours to delineate their nature, the presence of compression of the optic chiasm and any suprasellar or lateral extension of the tumour (a). A raised serum prolactin is typical of a pituitary tumour (b). A raised serum cyanate occurs in tobacco amblyopia (c). Bitemporal visual field defects result from any lesion that compresses the optic chiasm, including suprasellar meningiomas and giant anterior communicating artery aneurysms, as well as pituitary tumours (e).

Incorrect answers: d
The removal of a pituitary tumour is often followed by a rapid, even dramatic, improvement in visual acuity.

7. (see sections 4 and 18)

Correct answers: b, d
Subarachnoid haemorrhage associated with a third nerve palsy suggests posterior communicating artery aneurysm (b). A painful third nerve palsy, usually with a normal pupillary light reaction, may complicate diabetes mellitus due to infarction in the nerve (d).

Incorrect answers: a, c, e
The pupillomotor fibres are close to the surface of the third nerve and may be preferentially affected by compressive lesions such as posterior communicating artery aneurysms such that the pupil is dilated and unreactive. In diabetes and other conditions causing infarcts within the third nerve, the pupil is often spared. However, pupil sparing does not necessarily exclude a compressive lesion (a). Although a cause of headache and diplopia and headache, temporal arteritis (Fig. 196) is extremely rare in young adults and is not associated with meningism (c). Migrainous neuralgia is not a cause of a third nerve palsy (e).

8.

Correct answers: a
The left hemisphere is likely to be dominant (containing the speech centre) even in left handed patients. As such, progressive dysphasia should always suggest a left hemisphere lesion.

Incorrect answers: b, c, d, e
Dressing dyspraxia is a feature of non-dominant (right) hemisphere lesions (b). Seizures with head turning to the left suggest a right hemisphere lesion (c). Spastic dysarthria as in motor neuron disease is due to bilateral lesion (d). Wasting and weakness are due to a lower motor neuron lesion, e.g. lumbar disc disease, not a hemisphere lesion (e).

9. (see sections 25, 26, 30 and 31)

Correct answers: a, b
Patients with diabetes mellitus frequently show wasting of their intrinsic hand muscles. This may be due to nerve palsies, e.g. median or ulnar nerve palsies, or as part of a generalized diabetic peripheral neuropathy (a). Wasting of hand muscles occurs in patients with hereditary motor and sensory neuropathy (HMSN) (b).

Incorrect answers: c, d, e
It is uncommon for intrinsic hand muscles (T1) to be wasted in cervical spondylosis, which most frequently affects higher levels of the cervical spine (C5–7) (c). Wasting of intrinsic hand muscles is uncommon in dermatomyositis, which usually affects proximal rather than distal muscles (d). In cerebral palsy the hand may appear small, not due to muscle wasting, but to poor development of the affected limb (e).

10. (see section 27)

Correct answers: a, d, e
A positive response to a short-acting anticholinesterase (e.g. edrophonium, the Tensilon test) is diagnostic of myasthenia gravis, (a). On muscle sampling, jitter is a characteristic feature of myasthenia (d). IVig is the treatment of choice in severe uncontrolled myasthenia gravis (e). Steroids are also useful.

Incorrect answers: b, c
When steroid treatment is started it is important that only small doses are given as in some cases steroids may result in a dramatic initial increased weakness. In patients already treated with anticholinesterases, intravenous edrophonium may be hazardous (b). In these cases edrophonium should only be administered in hospital and only a small dose should be used because of the risk of provoking a cholinergic crisis (c).

11. (see section 24)

Correct answers: a, b, c, d, e
The majority of newly diagnosed people with Parkinson's disease, with akinesia, will respond to L-dopa. Failure to do so questions the clinical diagnosis. Patients with parkinsonism rather than Parkinson's disease may also fail to respond to L-dopa (a). The peripheral effects of L-dopa may result in postural hypotension (b). Lewy body disease is characterized by visual hallucinations and dementia together with some parkinsonian features (c). Of the principal features of Parkinson's disease, namely tremor, rigidity and akinesia, tremor is the least responsive to L-dopa (d). Akinesia is the most disabling feature of Parkinson's disease (e).

12. (see section 35)

Correct answers: a, b, e
Vitamin B$_{12}$ deficiency is an important treatable cause of dementia (a). The Herxheimer reaction may complicate therapy of tertiary syphilis with penicillin. It can be avoided by pre-treating the patient with steroids prior to administering penicillin (b). Cholinergic drugs, including the anticholinesterases donepezil (Aricept) and rivastigmine (Exelon), slow progression of dementia in patients with Alzheimer's disease (e).

Incorrect answers: c, d
When treating hypothyroidism, particularly in the elderly, it is important to begin treatment with small doses of thyroxine to avoid precipitating cardiac failure (c). There are no specific CSF abnormalities in Alzheimer's disease (d).

13. (see sections 4, 5, 27)

Correct answers: a, b, c, d, e
Monocular diplopia is virtually never due to neurological disease (a). A sixth nerve palsy with lateral rectus weakness results in double vision with side-to-side separation of the images on lateral gaze to the side of the weak muscle (b). Myasthenia is an important cause of double vision (c). In binocular diplopia the outer image is always the false image (d). Because of its long course within the skull, sixth nerve palsy is not a reliable localizing sign (it may be a false localizing sign) (e).

14. (see section 8)

Correct answers: a, b, c, d, e
In Bell's palsy hyperacusis is due to involvement of the nerve to stapedius (a). An additional sixth nerve palsy suggests a lesion within the brainstem (b). An absent corneal reflex suggests a lesion in the cerebello-pontine angle (c). Crocodile tears are a long-term complication of Bell's palsy (d). Lyme disease should be considered in patients from southern Germany and Austria, and from southern England (e).

15. (see section 14)

Correct answers: c, d
This patient has amaurosis fugax. On fundoscopic examination cholesterol emboli may be visible, particularly at points of bifurcation of the fundal arterioles (c). The patient is likely to have bilateral carotid stenoses and with left-sided amaurosis she is at risk of an embolus occluding her left middle cerebral artery resulting in dysphasia and a right hemiplegia (d).

Incorrect answers: a, b, e
Although aspirin is usually the drug of choice in amaurosis fugax, this patient has atrial fibrillation and therefore should be anticoagulated with warfarin prior to cardioversion (a). Transient unilateral blindness frequently occurs from emboli originating from carotid stenosis. It is not due to vascular disease in vertebrobasilar territory (b). Endarterectomy is only indicated if a carotid stenosis exceeds 70%. Below this the risks of surgery are greater than the risks from medical management (e).

16. (see section 21)

Correct answers: a, b
This patient has late-onset focal epilepsy. In the United Kingdom the doctor may notify the vehicle licensing authority if the patient fails to do so (a). With olfactory hallucinations there is a strong possibility of finding a structural abnormality in the temporal lobe on an MRI scan (b).

Incorrect answers: c, d, e
Although an EEG may be abnormal, an MRI is the most important investigation in demonstrating a possible intracranial tumour (c). If a meningioma presents with epilepsy, after its removal the patient is still at risk of seizures (d). Phenytoin is not the first-line anticonvulsant of choice. Although an effective anticonvulsant, it has a limited dose range which, when exceeded, frequently causes drug intoxication (e).

17. (see section 32)

Correct answers: a, b, d, e
This patient has communicating hydrocephalus presenting with a triad of dementia, gait disturbance and urinary incontinence. On CT or MR scanning dilatation of the ventricles without evidence of cerebral atrophy is typical of a communicating hydrocephalus (a). Improvement of gait following the removal of a large volume of CSF suggests the patient will respond to ventriculo-peritoneal CSF shunting (b), leading particularly to improvement in gait (d). Communicating hydrocephalus may follow a trivial head injury (e).

Incorrect answers: c
Alzheimer's disease is not associated with a gait disturbance in its early stages.

18. (see section 21)

Correct answers: a, c, e
Absence attacks are not always obvious in children and this may affect educational performance (a). Hyperventilation may induce minor generalized seizures with spike and wave discharges during EEG recordings (c), which are diagnostic of petit mal (e).

Incorrect answers: b, d
Phenytoin is not the drug of choice in minor generalized epilepsy (b). Absence attacks frequently stop in later life (d).

19. (see section 36)

Correct answers: a, e
Any manoeuvre which would normally raise intracranial pressure, including straining, will worsen the headache of raised intracranial pressure (a). In raised intracranial pressure the optic disc margins may be blurred with the development of papilloedema (e).

Incorrect answers: b, c, d
Headache preceded by visual teichopsia suggests migraine rather than raised intracranial pressure (b). Scalp tenderness may suggest temporal arteritis (c). Neck stiffness suggests meningism rather than raised intracranial pressure (d).

20. (see section 31)

Correct answers: d
This patient has sciatica, most likely due to a prolapsed intervertebral lumbar disc. Bladder dysfunction associated with sciatica suggests central disc protrusion and is an indication for urgent imaging and surgery.

Incorrect answers: a, b, c, e
In root lesions including sciatica the pain is experienced in the relevant root distribution (a). With weakness of the right foot dorsiflexion, the prolapsed disc is most likely to involve L4. As such the ankle jerk will be preserved (b). Not all prolapsed intervertebral discs require surgery. Most can be successfully managed conservatively (c). The disc prolapse is expected at L5, not S1 (d).

21. (see section 26)

Correct answers: a, c, e
This patient has polymyositis. This may be a manifestation of an underlying occult malignancy (a). High-dose steroid therapy, with immunosuppressant drugs, is the treatment of choice in polymyositis (c). A rolling Trendelenburg gait due to weakness of pelvic girdle muscles is typical of primary muscle disease including polymyositis (e).

Incorrect answers: b, d
In polymyositis a muscle biopsy will demonstrate inflammatory, not atrophic changes (b). Muscle sampling at EMG will demonstrate myopathic abnormalities, often also with fibrillation potentials (d).

22. (see section 36)

Correct answers: c, d
This patient has classical migraine. Sudden onset of persistent weakness and dysphasia suggests an additional vascular lesion (in this case cerebral infarction) in her dominant left hemisphere (c). Beta-blockers are useful in reducing the frequency of migrainous headaches (d).

Incorrect answers: a, b, e
The combination of dysphasia and right hemiplegia results from a left-sided, not a right-sided cerebral lesion (a). Although haemorrhage may occur in cerebral metastases, this clinical history suggests vascular rather than malignant disease (b). Infrequently migraine may be symptomatic of intracranial lesions, particularly vascular anomalies such as arterio-venous malformations (e).

23. (see sections 30 and 32)

Correct answers: a, b, c, d
Downbeat nystagmus suggests a lesion at the cranio-cervical junction, most likely a Chiari type 1 malformation. This is frequently associated with syringomyelia, accounting for absent reflexes in the upper limbs and bilateral extensor plantar responses. Dissociated sensory loss in the upper limbs (loss of temperature sensation with preserved touch sensation) is typical of a central spinal cord lesion (a). Syringomyelia is frequently associated with hydrocephalus (b). Ataxia and incontinence also suggest hydrocephalus (c). Suspended sensory loss is also characteristic of a central spinal cord lesion (d).

Incorrect answers: e
Peripheral neuropathies are often associated with absent reflexes: however, absent reflexes restricted to the upper limbs suggest either extensive cervical root lesions or a central cervical spinal cord lesion.

24. (see section 20)

Correct answers: a, b, e
This man has acromegaly with prominent supra-orbital ridges (a). Compression of the optic chiasma with pituitary tumour causes bitemporal visual field defects (b). Acromegaly may be associated with a cardiomyopathy (e).

Incorrect answers: c, d
Acromegaly results from excessive growth hormone production from an acidophil adenoma of the pituitary (c). Carpal tunnel syndrome is a recognized complication of acromegaly, which occurs independently of any coexisting diabetes mellitus (d).

25. (see section 33)

Correct answers: a, b, e
This patient had an extradural haematoma. This is often associated with a temporary lucid interval before raised intracranial pressure and coma develop (a). The development of a third nerve palsy suggests transtentorial herniation (coning) causing the nerve to become compressed at the tentorial edge between the posterior cerebral and superior cerebellar arteries (b). Extradural haematoma is likely to be due to damage to the middle meningeal artery resulting from traumatic fracture of the skull (e).

Incorrect answers: c, d
The history and physical signs suggest a head injury rather than an injury to the cervical spine (c). The sixth nerve does not innervate the pupil. Pupillary dilation suggests a compressive lesion of the third nerve (d).

26. (see section 21)

Correct answers: a, d
This patient has focal seizures arising from a lesion in the right cerebral hemisphere. In patients with congenital lesions, including birth trauma or other cerebral lesions occurring before the end of the growth spurt, the affected limb may be smaller, not due to muscle wasting but because of incomplete development (a). An astrocytoma or any other intracerebral tumour in the right hemisphere could account for this patient's focal epilepsy (d).

Incorrect answers: b, c, e
Irrespective of a patient's age, focal epilepsy must always be fully investigated with MRI scanning, etc., to determine the presence of any structural lesion (b). Cerebral tumours can occur at any age. A meningioma is an important cause of epilepsy, but in this case the lesion was right sided (c). Although an effective anticonvulsant, phenytoin has a limited dose range which, if exceeded, frequently results in toxicity (e).

27. (see section 36)

Correct answers: b, c, d, e
This patient has temporal arteritis (Fig. 196). Double vision is a common complication of temporal arteritis (b). Patients with temporal arteritis frequently have muscular pains from coexisting polymyalgia rheumatica (c). With high-dose steroids, clinical improvement with a fall in the ESR occurs within 48 hours (d). Blindness may be a permanent complication (e).

Incorrect answers: a
Temporal artery biopsy is an important investigation of suspected temporal arteritis. However, the biopsy is frequently negative and the diagnosis is determined on clinical grounds with significant elevation of the ESR.

28. (see section 27)

Correct answers: a, c, d, e
This patient had the Lambert–Eaton myasthenic syndrome (LEMS) complicating a bronchogenic carcinoma. In myasthenia gravis tendon reflexes may fatigue (a). Thyroid dysfunction, particularly thyrotoxicosis, may result in a dramatic deterioration in patients with myasthenia gravis (c). Anti-MUSK antibodies may be present in myasthenic patients especially if acetylcholine receptor antibodies are not detectable (d). In LEMS the tendon reflexes are frequently sluggish or absent, but increase following sustained muscle contraction (e).

Incorrect answers: b
Double vision is unusual in the Lambert–Eaton syndrome but common in myasthenia gravis.

29. (see section 30)

Correct answers: a, c, d, e
This man has lumbar canal stenosis. In some cases the neurological examination at rest may be normal, but abnormal signs, absent reflexes, sensory loss or even weakness may be elicited if the patient is re-examined after exercise (a). The ankle reflexes (S1) are not compromised in a patient with a prolapsed intervertebral disc at L4 (c). Symptomatic lumbar canal stenosis often responds well to surgical decompression, but back pain itself is often not relieved (d). Arterio-venous malformations of the spinal cord may also cause pain and weakness of the lower limbs on exercise (e).

Incorrect answers: b
Patients with lumbar canal stenosis may have little difficulty in climbing stairs, as this involves flexion of the lumbar spine, increasing the anterior–posterior diameter of the lumbar spine thus reducing pressure on the cauda equina. Therefore, if patients with suspected lumbar canal stenosis are to be examined after exercise, it is important that they are exercised on the flat.

30. (see section 21)

Correct answers: a, b, e
Myoclonus typically occurs in metabolic disorders such as Gaucher's disease (a), subacute sclerosing panencephalitis (SSPE) (b), and also in Creutzfeldt–Jakob disease, a prion disorder (e). It also occurs in idiopathic epilepsy.

Incorrect answers: c, d
Myoclonus is not a feature of diabetes or motor neuron disease.

31. (see section 25)

Correct answers: b, c, d, e
This patient has meralgia paraesthetica caused by compression of the lateral cutaneous nerve of the thigh as it passes beneath the inguinal ligament in the groin, and a peripheral neuropathy (b). Meralgia paraesthetica may be a presentation of diabetes (c). An absent sural sensory action potential is typical of a peripheral neuropathy (d). Injection of anaesthetic into the lateral femoral cutaneous nerve may leave irritating numbness in the outer thigh (e).

Incorrect answers: a
This patient's symptoms are not caused by a disc prolapse.

32. (see section 3)

Correct answers: c, d
This patient has a myotonic pupil. Absent reflexes in the lower limbs are often found (the Holmes–Adie syndrome) (c). The myotonic pupil eventually contracts to a sustained light stimulus (d).

Incorrect answers: a, b, e
Without other features a third nerve palsy can be excluded. Horner's syndrome is due to damage to the sympathetic innervation to the dilator pupillae muscle. A myotonic pupil may occur without areflexia in the lower limbs.

33. (see section 24)

Correct answers: a, b, c, e
Postural tremor may be induced by a variety of drugs including salbutamol and sodium valproate (a). The tremor of Parkinson's disease is usually asymmetrical (b). Beta-blockers may be useful in the treatment of benign essential tremor (c). Tremors and other movement disorders may follow treatment with neuroleptic drugs, for example phenothiazines (e).

Incorrect answers: d
Parkinsonian tremor responds, but only partially, to L-dopa and dopa agonists.

34. (see section 10)

Correct answers: a, b, c, d
Nausea and vomiting are frequent with peripheral vertigo (a). Additional
dysarthria and weakness of the limbs would suggest vertebrobasilar ischaemia (b).
Vertigo on neck extension is regarded as a feature of cervical spondylosis (c).

Incorrect answers: e
Cawthorne–Epley exercises are useful in suppressing peripheral not central
vertigo.

35.

Correct answers: b, d
This patient has diabetic amyotrophy and a peripheral neuropathy. A blood
sugar estimation is an important investigation (b). Diabetic amyotrophy is due
to diabetic lumbar plexopathy (diabetic proximal motor neuropathy) (d).

Incorrect answers: a, c, e
Prolapsed intervertebral disc prolapse can be painless. Extension of the knee is
relatively preserved in a pyramidal (UMN) lesion affecting the leg. An L4/5
prolapsed disc would result in wasting of the anterior tibial compartment, not
the thigh.

36.

Correct answers: a, c, d, e
Myxoedema may be associated with ataxia of gait (the cerebellar syndrome of
hypothyroidism) (a), deafness (c), dementia (d), and psychosis ('myxoedemic
madness') (e).

Incorrect answers: b
Hypothyroidism is associated with menorrhagia, not amenorrhoea.

37. (see section 25)

Correct answers: a, c
This man has a hereditary motor and sensory neuropathy (HMSN). Slowing of
conduction velocity is characteristic of demyelinating peripheral neuropathies
(a). Preservation of tendon reflexes suggests an axonal neuropathy (c).

Incorrect answers: b, d, e
Immunosuppression does not influence the clinical course of HSMN. Type 2
HSMN is due to an axonal, not a demyelinating neuropathy. HSMN type 1 is
due to a demyelinating neuropathy. There are many different mutations causing
these clinical syndromes.

38. (see section 34)

Correct answers: b, c, d
The oculo-cephalic reflex may be abolished in sedated patients (b). In the unconscious patient, deviation of the eyes towards the side of stimulus when ice-cold water is infused in the ear (cold opposite, warm same: COWS) denotes continuing brainstem activity (c). When testing for irreversible brain damage, it is essential that the patient is not hypothermic (d).

Incorrect answers: a, e
When ice-cold water is instilled into the ear of an unconscious patient, tonic deviation of the eyes and not nystagmus is seen if brainstem activity is functioning. Nystagmus requires consciousness.

39.

Correct answers: a, b, c, d
This patient has trigeminal neuralgia. If the patient is allergic to carbamazepine, other anticonvulsants may be effective (a). An absent corneal response suggests a lesion at the cerebello-pontine angle (b). The mandibular and maxillary divisions of the nerve are usually affected in trigeminal neuralgia (c). Trigeminal neuralgia may occur in younger patients with multiple sclerosis (d).

Incorrect answers: e
Trigeminal neuralgia is not a complication of diabetes.

40.

Correct answers: a, b, c, e
The CSF glucose is characteristically low in malignant meningitis (a). The CSF glucose is also low in bacterial meningitis (b). In general, a lumbar puncture should not be performed (b) without ensuring the CT scan is normal, for fear of coning (c), but start treatment while preparing for the scan and LP. Cryptococcal meningitis may complicate immune deficiency disorders (e).

Incorrect answers: d
A purpuric rash suggests meningococcal rather than *Haemophilus* meningitis.

41.

Correct answers: a, b, e
Beta-interferon slows acquisition of disability in relapsing remitting multiple sclerosis (a). Multiple sclerosis may present with a progressive spastic paraparesis (b). Patients with multiple sclerosis may deteriorate transiently on exercise (Uthoff's phenomenon) (e).

Incorrect answers: c, d
Beta-interferon may reduce the frequency of relapses but it has less effect on the eventual disability.

42.

Correct answers: a
This patient has narcolepsy. Nocturnal sleep is typically interrupted in narcolepsy.

Incorrect answers: b, c, d, e
Dream recall is better if a patient is woken during REM sleep than during deep stage 4 sleep. Sleep paralysis is an accessory symptom of narcolepsy and is not epileptic. In narcolepsy, collapse evoked by strong emotion is due to cataplexy, not hysteria. The accessory symptoms of narcolepsy, including cataplexy and sleep paralysis, respond poorly to dexamfetamine.

43.

Correct answers: b
Progressive ataxia can be a presentation of an occult malignancy (b).

Incorrect answers: a, c, d, e
This patient is too old to have Friedreich's ataxia. Addison's disease is not associated with ataxia. Hypo- not hyperthyroidism is associated with ataxia. An MRI scan is essential in the investigation of ataxia, particularly to exclude neoplasm.

44.

Correct answers: b, e
Non-metastatic manifestations of malignant disease include a predominantly sensory neuropathy (b) and painful muscle weakness (polymyositis) (e).

Incorrect answers: a, c, d
Amyotrophic lateral sclerosis, spinal cord compression and myasthenia gravis are not non-metastatic manifestations of malignant disease.

45.

Correct answers: a, d, e
A high CSF protein with no accompanying cellular increase occurs in spinal cord compression (Froin's syndrome) (a), acoustic neurinoma (d) and Guillain–Barré syndrome (e).

Incorrect answers: b, c
In tuberculosis and meningococcal meningitis the CSF protein is frequently elevated, but this is accompanied by a cellular increase in the spinal fluid.

46.

Correct answers: a, b, e
Bitemporal hemianopsia due to compression of the optic chiasm can occur in craniopharyngioma (a) and pituitary adenoma (b). Apparent bitemporal visual field defects due to centro-caecal scotomas may occur in patients with tobacco amblyopia (e).

Incorrect answers: c, d
Left temporal lesions would cause an homonymous right upper quadrantic defect and not a bitemporal field defect. A posterior communicating artery (PICA) aneurysm is not associated with a visual field defect.

47.

Correct answers: a, c, e
This patient has developed right carotid dissection following trauma to her neck. A Horner's syndrome strongly suggests a dissection of the internal carotid artery (a). An MRA study is important in investigating a suspected carotid occlusion (c). Anticoagulation with warfarin is the treatment of choice in carotid artery dissection (e).

Incorrect answers: b, d
The clinical history is that of trauma, not long-standing migraine. A normal CT scan does not exclude a carotid dissection. MRI and MRA are more reliable investigations.

48.

Correct answers: a, c, d
This man has sustained a subarachnoid haemorrhage. Hydrocephalus is a common complication of a subarachnoid haemorrhage (a). Confusion and lower limb weakness suggest vascular spasm in anterior cerebral artery territory (c). Cerebral aneurysms may be familial (d).

Incorrect answers: b, e
A third nerve palsy suggests a posterior communicating (PCommA) and not an anterior communicating artery (ACommA) aneurysm. Large aneurysms >10 mm in diameter are thought to pose less risk of haemorrhage.

49.

Correct answers: b, c
This man has dementia. Small unreacting pupils (possible Argyll Robertson pupils) and a neuropathic ankle joint suggest neurosyphilis (b). HIV testing is important as AIDS can result in dementia (c).

Incorrect answers: a, d, e
Nystagmus and absent ankle jerks suggest Wernicke's encephalopathy. Thyrotoxicosis is not a cause of dementia. Cholinergic drugs (anticholinesterases), not anticholinergic drugs, may be important in the treatment of Alzheimer's disease.

50.

Correct answers: b, c, e
This man has a non-dominant hemisphere tumour. Dressing apraxia suggests a non-dominant parietal lesion (b). Additional dysphasia would suggest cerebral metastases (c). However, the progressive history suggests a right hemisphere tumour (e).

Incorrect answers: a, d
The progressive history suggests tumour rather than cerebral infarction. Headaches are more likely to be due to raised intracranial pressure than temporal arteritis.

Index